# MANAGED CARE

## and Children With Special Health Care Needs

American Academy of Pediatrics
PO Box 927
141 Northwest Point Blvd
Elk Grove Village, IL 60009-0927

Library of Congress Catalog Card No. 97-073373

ISBN No. 0-910761-89-2

MA0104

Prices on request. Address all inquiries to:
American Academy of Pediatrics, PO Box 927, 141 Northwest Point Blvd, Elk Grove Village,
IL 60009-0927.

The recommendations in this publication do not indicate an exclusive course of treatment or serve as a standard of medical care. Variations, taking into account individual circumstances, may be appropriate.

Printed in the United States of America.

## Project Advisory Committee for the Medical Home Program for Children With Special Needs: 1994–1998

Calvin Sia, MD, *Chairperson*
Gilbert A. Buchanan, MD
Antoinette Eaton, MD
Arthur Lavin, MD
John A. Nackashi, MD
Judith Palfrey, MD
John R. Poncher, MD

## Committee on Child Health Financing: 1996–1997

Stephen Berman, MD, *Chairperson*
Joseph C. Bogdan, MD
John S. Curran, MD
Arthur Garson, Jr, MD
Neal Halfon, MD, MPH
Robert Kay, MD
Beverly L. Koops, MD
Maria E. Minon, MD
Richard P. Nelson, MD

## Committee on Children With Disabilities: 1996–1997

Philip R. Ziring, MD, *Chairperson*
Dana Brazdziunas, MD
Lilliam González de Pijem, MD
Robert LaCamera, MD
John R. Poncher, MD
Richard D. Quint, MD, MPH
Virginia F. Randall, MD
Elizabeth Ruppert, MD
Adrian D. Sandler, MD

## Contributing Editor

Margaret McManus

## Staff Editors

Dorit Naftalin
Elizabeth Osterhus
Thomas Tonniges, MD
Edward Zimmerman

# INTRODUCTION

The American Academy of Pediatrics (AAP) believes that all children should have a medical home where health care services are accessible, family-centered, continuous, comprehensive, coordinated, compassionate, and culturally competent. The physician and the family are jointly accountable for the medical home. For children with special needs it is particularly important to have a medical home. The changing health care environment and the increasing presence of managed care pose both challenges and opportunities to ensuring that children with special health care needs and their families have access to appropriate medical care.

To address these concerns, we are pleased to offer you this compendium, *Managed Care and Children With Special Health Care Needs.* The compendium has been developed as a joint project of the AAP Medical Home Program for Children With Special Needs (MHPCSN), the AAP Committee on Child Health Financing (COCHF), and the AAP Committee on Children With Disabilities (COCWD). Margaret McManus, President of McManus Health Policy, Inc., and consultant to COCHF, assisted the Committees in preparing the issue briefs. The goal of the MHPCSN is to develop materials that support pediatric providers who care for children with special needs in managed care arrangements. This program is funded by a 4-year grant (1994–1998) from the federal Maternal and Child Health Bureau (MCJ-17R003). The COCHF develops policy, resources, and information services on managed care for pediatricians and families, and policy statements on child health financing issues including Medicaid. The COCWD studies and develops policy on the role of pediatricians in the long-term outcome of children with chronic diseases and disabilities in relation to functional ability, psycho-

social adaptation, and vocational potential. The COCHF and COCWD also jointly address issues regarding the delivery of community-based health care services for dehospitalized, technology-dependent, and chronically ill children.

The materials in this packet are intended to assist all pediatric providers in understanding the issues that affect services for children with special needs and their families. Included in this packet are six issue briefs addressing topics that are of greatest concern to pediatricians and other providers caring for children with special heath care needs in a managed care environment. The issue briefs address the following:

- how to define and identify the population
- issues relating to gatekeeping, service authorization, and profiling
- the use of capitation and risk adjustment
- strategies of care coordination
- what constitutes quality care
- approaches to integrated system designs

These issue briefs are supplemented by pertinent AAP policy statements and articles that describe effective strategies for providing service to children with special health care needs. [Please note that AAP policy statements are reviewed every 3 years by the authoring body, at which time a recommendation is made that the policy be retired, revised, or reaffirmed without change. (Status of the policy may be determined by contacting the Academy.)]

We thank you for your interest in children with special health care needs and for your efforts to advocate on their behalf.

# Table of Contents

# ISSUE
# BRIEFS

# DEFINING AND IDENTIFYING CHILDREN WHO HAVE SPECIAL HEALTH CARE NEEDS

## Problem Statement

Children with chronic conditions or disabilities are commonly described as having special health care needs. National studies show that from 20% to 30% of children have chronic conditions. Not only do these children require preventive and acute health care services, many also need additional health services as part of their initial identification and evaluation, intermittent and ongoing treatment, and daily routine care.

There is no uniformly accepted approach for identifying children with special health care needs because of the diversity of this population and the difficulties associated with defining severity and functional status. The conditions of children with developmental, behavioral, and emotional challenges are the most difficult to define. Consequently, managed care organizations and pediatric providers who assume medical responsibility including the financial responsibility for payment for these children who require higher cost care are often unable to anticipate their health care needs or develop appropriate risk-sharing arrangements.

The following set of issues highlights the key areas of concern pediatricians face when defining a child with special health care needs.

## Key Issues

• While there are several different approaches that can be used to identify children who have, or are at risk of having, chronic conditions, each approach has significant drawbacks. For example:

  *Condition or diagnostic approaches* are limited because they may be unwieldy and fail to distinguish severity, impairment, or service needs. Also, many rare conditions may be omitted from the conditions list, or would make the list inordinately long if they were included.

  *Functional status approaches* are limited because they may exclude children who function well but still need ongoing health services to maintain their function. Also, there are substantial problems in the measurement of children's function, given variations in their ages and stages of development.

  *Service-based approaches* are limited because they exclude children who may need, but do not use, services. Also, it is unclear what type or amount of health service is predictive of future patterns of care.

  *Public program eligibility approaches* — such as receipt of Supplemental Security Income (SSI), foster care assistance, or Title V services for children with special health care needs — are limited because these programs tend to exclude middle- and upper-income children and also children with less severe conditions.

  *Cost-based approaches* may be limited because many children with high costs may have short-term health problems and, in any given year, many children may not meet the cost trigger but still have ongoing chronic care needs.

• In Medicaid, SSI program eligibility is the most commonly used approach for identifying children with special needs. Many children who are AFDC-eligible, however, may also have special health care needs. Furthermore, SSI includes many children who have only minimal special health care needs.

• In private health insurance plans, there are no common approaches for prospectively identifying children with special health care needs. Rather, once enrolled, cost triggers and service utilization "outliers" are the most often used methods for identifying children with special health care needs, generally for the purpose of more aggressive care management.

3

## Summary of Approaches for Identifying Children With Special Health Care Needs

1. The Maternal and Child Health Bureau, in 1995, convened a Work Group on Defining Children with Special Health Care Needs. They developed the following definition for Title V agencies for the purpose of planning and systems development:

   Children with special health care needs are those who have or are at elevated risk for chronic physical, developmental, behavioral, or emotional conditions and who also require health and related services of a type or amount not usually required by children.[1]

   The continuum of services required to improve or maintain functioning includes specialized or enhanced medical and nursing services; therapeutic services; family support services; medical equipment and supplies; and related child care, early intervention and special education services, social services, and transportation.

2. The National Association of Children's Hospitals and Related Institutions in 1997 plans to release licensed software for the classification of childhood conditions.[2] Using ICD-9-CM diagnosis codes, the software will classify children by type of condition, severity, and disease progression. It is intended for use in tracking chronic disease prevalence within a plan or practice, profiling health service utilization, pricing and capitation risk adjustment, and tracking quality indicators.

3. The Social Security Administration has one of the only operational approaches for determining childhood disability.[3] More than 100 specific diagnoses that may disable children are listed. Since the passage of the Personal Responsibility and Work Opportunities Act, children are no longer eligible solely on the basis of a functional impairment.

4. Researchers at Albert Einstein College of Medicine have developed a new questionnaire for identifying children with chronic conditions, the Questionnaire for Identifying Children with Chronic Conditions (QuICCC).[4] The questionnaire asks about the specific consequences of having a chronic health condition related to functional limitations, reliance on compensatory mechanisms or assistance, and service use or need beyond that which is considered routine. A variation of this method has been used to identify children with chronic health conditions in the National Health Interview Survey Supplement on Disability.

5. Researchers at the New England Medical Center have developed a modified SF-36 health status questionnaire form for children, published in early 1997.[5] It is called the Child Health Questionnaire. The content of the Child Health Questionnaire addresses 14 dimensions: physical functioning, role/social-physical, general health perceptions, bodily pain, parental impact-time, parental impact-emotional, role/social-behavioral, self-esteem, mental health, general behavior, family activities, family cohesion, and change in health. (For information contact The Health Institute at the New England Medical Center, Box 345, 750 Washington St, Boston, MA 02111.)

## Implications for Practicing Pediatricians

There are two key principles that pediatricians may find useful in identifying children with special health care needs in their practices and managed care plans and defining their needs. First, no single definition will be acceptable to everyone. Using a combination of approaches to identify children with special needs is important. For example, diagnosis plus service volume or diagnosis plus functional status is preferable to relying on any single approach. Second, the diversity of the population of children with chronic conditions makes the need for flexibility and breadth of definition essential. For example, children who have a parent with mental illness may not have a chronic condition but may be at far greater risk of adverse health outcomes than children with a confirmed chronic condition. Similarly, children with a chronic condition and no functional impairment may require more services on an intermittent basis than children with functional limitation.

It is advisable to address the following issues as a critical step toward improving the identification of children with special needs:

- Determine the approach used by the state's Medicaid agency to define and reimburse plans serving children with special health care needs.

- Find out how managed care plans identify and differentiate children with special health care needs in terms of assigning primary care providers, setting risk-adjusted capitation methods, authorizing specialty pediatric services, providing case management, monitoring service utilization, and monitoring quality performance.

- Obtain information on how the administrative data systems at the payer, plan, and practice levels can be used to identify children with special health care needs.

- Ascertain what additional methods could be used to identify children with special needs; these might include new member assessments, special focused studies, use of existing SSI medical listings, and surveys that measure functional status.

- Recommend ways payers, managed care plans, and pediatric practices can achieve uniformity in the identification of children with special health care needs.

. . . . . . . . . . .

1. Maternal and Child Health Bureau: *Definition of Children with Special Health Care Needs.* Rockville, MD: Division of Services for Children With Special Health Care Needs; 1995
2. National Association of Children's Hospitals and Related Institutions. *Overview Presentation on NACHRI Classification of Congenital and Chronic Health Conditions: Purposes and Uses, Structure, Definitions, and Illustrations.* Alexandria, VA: National Association of Children's Hospitals and Related Institutions, May 10, 1996
3. National Commission on Childhood Disability. *Supplemental Security Income for Children With Disabilities.* Washington, DC: National Commission on Childhood Disability; 1995
4. Stein REK, Westbrook LE, Bauman LJ.: The Questionnaire for Identifying Children with Chronic Conditions (QuICCC): a measure based on a noncategorical approach. *Pediatrics* (to be published)
5. Landgraf JM, Abetz LN, Ware J. *Child Health Questionnaire (CHQ): a user's manual.* Boston, MA: The Health Institute at the New England Medical Center; 1996

# GATEKEEPING, SERVICE AUTHORIZATION, AND PROFILING

## Problem Statement

Pediatricians are being asked to assume greater responsibilities for managing and authorizing the use of a broad range of health services, including specialty services, diagnostic tests and procedures, hospital services, and more. With this added responsibility comes new financial and performance incentives to control the use of health services and to meet certain quality-of-care requirements. In fact, pediatricians are one of the most profiled group of physicians, possibly because they serve a comparatively healthy population compared to physicians serving adults.[1]

Several factors influence the ability of pediatricians and other primary care providers to assume these new functions:

- Their involvement in developing service authorization and profiling policies

- The efficiency and flexibility of service authorization

- The training of utilization review staff in pediatric care

- The adequacy of pediatric specialty networks within managed care plans

- The extent of case-mix adjustments

- The existing research and medical consensus on the effectiveness of various pediatric interventions

- The extent of discretion associated with medical necessity determinations and parents' knowledge regarding prior approval requirements

If these management systems are not fairly and efficiently structured, adversarial problems can result among pediatricians and managed care plans, among general pediatricians and pediatric medical subspecialists and pediatric surgical specialists, and among families and pediatricians.

The following set of issues highlights the key areas of concern pediatricians encounter in gatekeeping, service authorization, and profiling.*

## Key Issues

- Profiling is typically based on claims data and often does not take into account case severity. Also, profiling data seldom control for physician specialty and do not distinguish between the referring physician and the physician providing the service. Unadjusted profiling data may adversely affect participating gatekeepers serving children with special needs.

- Primary care providers are assuming substantial financial and potential malpractice risk because of their obligation to manage all of the patient's care.

- Gatekeeping and service authorization systems can result in delays in appropriate referrals and treatment and produce adverse health outcomes and family dissatisfaction with access and quality of care.

- Ethical dilemmas associated with the use of financial incentives for decreasing service utilization are significant.

- A certain subset of children with complex health conditions may be most appropriately managed by experienced pediatricians practicing in a defined

* * * * * * * * * * *

* A *gatekeeper* (or care coordinator) is typically a primary care physician who is responsible for directly providing primary patient care as well as coordination of overall care. The gatekeeper determines the need for, and may authorize referrals to, specialists, use of certain tests, therapies, procedures, and admission to hospitals. Gatekeeping is predominantly a fiscal case management tool.

*Service authorization* requires permission from the gatekeeper and/or insurer before a patient can receive a particular type of medical or therapeutic service, be referred to a specialist, visit an emergency room, or be admitted to the hospital, in order for the service to be eligible for payment by the managed care plan.

*Profiling* is usually an assessment of health care economic efficiency based on analysis of patterns of care. Profiling may identify overutilization and underutilization of health care services, target ways of improving quality of care, and assess provider performance. Profiling typically demonstrates the relative statistical performance of a physician in relation to peers in terms of charges and service use.

area of expertise or by pediatric medical subspecialists, but with assurance of adequate primary care services.

- The effects of various gatekeeping systems have seldom been researched and, in some instances, may actually increase the cost of health. Restricted formularies have recently been shown to result in higher outpatient and inpatient utilization.

- Current graduate medical education training programs in pediatrics provide limited, if any, training in fiscal case management.

## Implications for the Practicing Pediatrician

There are several issues that pediatricians should consider as they assume greater clinical and financial responsibility under managed care.

- Develop an understanding of the scope of services that is included in the gatekeeper function and the types of financial incentives used.

- Become aware at the outset of the plan's panel of pediatric medical subspecialists, pediatric surgical specialists, and hospitals specializing in the care of children along with the plan's restrictions on the use of out-of-network pediatric providers.

- Examine the service authorization procedures used by the plan for other pediatric services including therapies, home care, formularies, durable medical equipment, and mental health services.[2]

- Examine carefully each plan's medical necessity guidelines that form the basis for service authorization decisions to assure that they take into account the unique developmental, rehabilitative, and habilitative needs of children. For Medicaid-insured children, there should be a broader interpretation of medical necessity than for children covered by commercial health insurance (consistent with the Early and Periodic Screening, Diagnosis, and Treatment [EPSDT] Program requirements.)[3, 4]

- Develop an understanding of the plan's methods for collecting and analyzing physician-specific health data.[5] It is critical for pediatricians to determine how the plan adjusts its profiling data and compares physician profiles to take into account those who serve a disproportionate share of children with special health care needs.

- Become actively involved in developing and reviewing physician-specific health care data as well as creating safeguards to prevent the unauthorized use of profiling data.

- Become aware of the possible perils associated with gatekeeping due to the increased liability exposure in managed care contracts: limits on care, financial incentives, care coordination (eg, potential liability for failed follow-up of referred patients), referral restrictions, practice scope, and plan exemptions. To avoid these problems, read your contract carefully and follow up with the patients.

1. Emmons DW, Wozniak GD. *Profiles and Feedback: Who Measures Physician Performance?* Chicago, IL: AMA; 1994

2. American Academy of Pediatrics, Committee on Child Health Financing. Guiding principles for managed care arrangements for the health care of infants, children, adolescents, and young adults. *Pediatrics.* 1995;95:613–615

3. Jameson E, Wehr E. Drafting national health care reform legislation to protect the health interest of children. *Stanford Law and Policy Review.* 1993;26:152–176

4. Fox HB, McManus MA. *Medicaid Managed Care for Children With Chronic or Disabling Conditions: Improved Strategies for States and Plans.* Washington, DC: Fox Health Policy Consultants, 1996

5. American Medical Association. *Physician Profiling and the Release of Physician-Specific Health Care Data.* Chicago, IL: AMA; 1995

# CAPITATION AND RISK ADJUSTMENT

## Problem Statement

The use of capitation allows for some flexibility in providing health services and a greater level of financial risk on the part of physicians and managed care plans. Currently, many pediatricians are capitated for just the routine primary and preventive services that they provide in their offices. A growing number, however, are being capitated for services that may include specialty and hospital care. Receiving fixed monthly payments per child may create inherent incentives to reduce the use of costly health care services.

Various risk adjustment methods are currently being used by state Medicaid agencies to account for differences in health needs. Few employers, however, adjust for risk. Most risk adjustment mechanisms have been developed for the elderly and adults with disabilities. Unfortunately, no valid or reliable pediatric risk adjustment approaches currently exist. As a result, adverse selection can result and children with high-cost conditions and their pediatric providers may be discriminated against in fully capitated arrangements. In addition, significant financial burdens on pediatric providers and restricted access to pediatric medical subspecialists, pediatric surgical specialists, and hospitals specializing in the care of children are likely to worsen unless appropriate capitation and risk adjustment methods can be developed.

The following set of issues highlights the key areas of concern pediatricians encounter in capitation and risk adjustment.

## Key Issues

- An increasing number of Medicaid children receiving Social Security Insurance (SSI) benefits and foster care assistance are enrolling in fully capitated managed care arrangements. Mandatory enrollment of American Families With Dependent Children (AFDC) children into Health Maintenance Organizations (HMOs) is becoming the norm.

- Considerable confusion exists regarding the managed care plan's and the physician's responsibility for delivering some or all of the Medicaid benefits in capitated managed care arrangements.

- The distribution of risk across plans and physicians is not random. Pediatricians are more likely to care for children with chronic conditions than are other primary care practitioners.

- Pediatricians in solo or small group practices may not be well positioned to move quickly into capitation. Also, pediatric medical subspecialists may have limited experience with this form of reimbursement.

- Medicaid capitation rates are typically set at 95% of the fee-for-service average by age, gender, or region. Since Medicaid's historic fee-for-service rates are so low, capitation rates can serve as a further disincentive to pediatricians' participation.

- Existing risk adjustment methods have limitations for children.

    Historic utilization and expenditures can be problematic for newborns and those who may need, but do not use, health services (eg, large numbers of children receiving SSI benefits have no prior utilization experience). Also, prior utilization may not take into account improved approaches for treatment.

    Age is problematic in that an insufficient number of breakdowns may be used for children (eg, under and over age 6; under and over age 18).

    Geographic area is problematic in that very poor, inner-city areas and rural areas may not be adequately taken into account.

    The SSI and foster care Medicaid eligibility categories are problematic in that huge variation in health service utilization exists within these categories. Also, many children receiving AFDC have significant health problems.

- Only recently has attention been focused on risk adjustment methods that take into account diagnosis. Use of diagnostic adjustments may be problematic, however, because of variations in severity and resource intensity within diagnoses. Also, certain ambulatory diagnoses are inconsistently coded among physicians and gaming of diagnoses may occur, as with the diagnostic related groups or DRGs. Privacy protections are another consideration.

- Attempting to capture functional status in risk adjustment methods may be too difficult to obtain.

- In more mature managed care markets, there is a need to determine how best to set and adjust future year payments when fee-for-service data become less available and predictable.

- Few positive incentives have been built into capitation to reward managed care plans and pediatricians who effectively and efficiently serve children with chronic conditions.

- Capitation arrangements and methods are changing at a fast pace.

- The use of capitation requires extensive oversight and evaluation as well as the ability to make timely refinements.

## Summary of Approaches for Capitation and Risk Adjustment for Children With Special Health Care Needs

1. *The Medicaid Working Group* is collaborating with several states, including Michigan, Missouri, New York, Ohio, and Wisconsin to develop clinical care models, reimbursement, and risk-sharing approaches for persons with disabilities.[1] Most of their work has focused on adults with disabilities, although a few new efforts are underway for children, as follows.

   In Ohio, SSI enrollees, excluding those with serious mental illness or mental retardation, are classified into one of seven different reimbursement levels based on prior claims data.[1] For example, plans would receive a monthly capitation of $165 for those with annual medical expenditures under $1,000; increasing in stages to $1,051 if expenditures were between $10,000 and $20,000. A new

single rate has been established for enrollees without any Medicaid claims history. Plans are then responsible for 90% of the first 5% profit or loss. For the next 10%, state and plans split savings and losses 50-50; for savings or losses greater than 15%, the state assumes 90% of the risk. Three HMOs partnering with academic medical centers were selected to implement these 2-year demonstration projects, called Accessing Better Care (ABC): United Health Care of Ohio, InHealth (with Columbus Children's Hospital), and HMO Health Ohio.

   In Wisconsin, SSI enrollees, aged 15 years and older, are classified into one of three cost groups based on prior Medicaid claims history and a blended single rate is developed.[1] The newly formed managed care plan serving this population (The Center for Independent Living) will assume risk for only the first 2% of costs above the capitated rate. It will also be allowed savings at the same rate.

   In Missouri, a new diagnostic-based system of risk adjustment is under development for SSI recipients.[2] More than 1,200 codes were initially judged as chronic conditions. Codes that showed statistically significant effects on expenditures were retained and those lacking effect were dropped or grouped together with other codes. Risk-sharing arrangements are being negotiated.

2. The *Managed Risk Medical Insurance Board* (MRMIB) has developed a risk adjustment method to reimburse 24 small group health insurance plans participating in the Health Insurance Plan of California.[3] The MRMIB is testing a health risk assessment and adjustment method for competing health plans. They have examined diagnoses with higher than average costs (more than $15,000), excluding normal maternity, mental health, chemical dependency, and trauma cases. Plans are given a ranking based on the number of high-cost patients served along with gender, family size, and age. A risk transfer among plans occurs when a plan exceeds the average cost by 5%. Plans with high outlier costs receive transfer funds from the lowest risk health plans. In their second year of testing, some revisions have been made to the rating system and money transfers. No information has yet been published on these revisions.

3. *Johns Hopkins School of Hygiene and Public Health* is developing a new pediatric risk adjustment system based on costs and diagnosis. Previously, Hopkins researchers, with the National Association of Children's Hospitals and Related Institutions, critically examined risk adjustment methods for children. [4] The new study's objective is to evaluate how well claims-based capitation adjustments reflect the true costs of the pediatric population. Use and expenditure data from children in the Maryland Medicaid program and children enrolled in a nonprofit health maintenance organization in Minnesota were used to test the following capitation adjustment models — Demographic, Diagnostic Cost Groups (DCGs), Payment Amounts for Capitated Systems (PACs), and Ambulatory Care Groups (ACGs). The authors found that even with the application of one of the capitation adjustment methods they evaluated, there was a significant underpayment for high-risk children. They concluded that any one of these is better than age and gender alone, but still substantial underprediction of risk remains.

4. The *Alameda County, California Committee on Children With Special Needs* is currently developing a pilot project to serve Medi-Cal children with special health care needs. They have devised a cumulative risk factor model for enhanced capitation rates — based on family and medical risk and agency involvement (Alameda County Committee on Children With Special Needs, Providing Health Care for Children With Special Needs in a Managed Care Environment, August 1994). The family risk factors include, but are not limited to, homeless (scoring 3), foster care (2), and teenage parents (2). The medical risk factors include very low birth weight (2), failure to thrive (1), and chronic medical problems (1 per problem). Agency involvement includes school Individual Education Plan (IEP) (1), infant program (1), regional center (1), and child protection services (1). A retrospective chart review of 1,500 patients was conducted using this model and approximately 10% of this sample scored 4 or more points. In the future, the committee recommends that such a checklist should be used as patients enter the practice or as their health or family status changes.

## Implications for Practicing Pediatricians

Several principles can help guide pediatricians as they enter into risk-based contracting. First, risk adjustment mechanisms should be constructed at the purchaser and plan levels to remove financial disincentives to care for children with special health care needs. Also, at the practice level, it is essential to even out the risks among all physicians, hospitals, and other health care providers. Until a pediatric risk adjustment approach has been tested and widely used, consider carve-outs for the child subgroups with very high-cost care and partial capitation combined with reinsurance and/or risk pools. Service carve-outs in addition or instead of population carve-outs might also be considered. These often include mental health services, health-related special education, and early intervention.[5] Other services that might be reimbursed on a fee-for-service basis include intensive ancillary therapies, durable medical equipment, and EPSDT expanded services. Second, the degree of risk assumed should be dependent on the number of enrollees in the managed care plan. The smaller the plan, the greater the need for risk-sharing mechanisms. Third, enhanced capitation rates provided to managed care plans for serving special-needs children should be reflected in higher payment levels to physicians. Pediatricians should determine what their state's Medicaid capitation rate is for SSI (oftentimes 2 or more times higher) and negotiate with the plan for the same rate. Oftentimes adjusted rates are not passed on to the pediatricians managing the child's care and too much financial risk is transferred to the primary care physician. However, until a sound empirically based risk adjustment mechanism is available, pediatricians should insist that they should receive fee-for-service payment for providing health care to chronically ill children. Another option is to negotiate an enhanced capitation rate.

The following additional information should be obtained before entering into risk-based contracting.

- Identify the specific services included in the capitated contract and determine which are exempted. The Academy's manual *A Pediatrician's Guide to Managed Care*[6] contains a comprehensive discussion on evaluating capitation rates.

- Determine the captitation rates set for children and the mechanisms used to adjust for chronic or disabling conditions. Learn if any adjustments are made for age, gender, geographic location, health status or diagnoses, and elevated use of health services.

- Ensure that stop-loss arrangements are available and how they come into play.

- Find out if any bonuses and withhold arrangements are used by the plan. Determine if they include any performance-based incentives for serving children with special health care needs.

1. *Medicaid Working Group Update.* Boston: Medicaid Working Group, November 1995.
2. Kronick R, Dreyfus T, Zhou A, and Lee L, *Risk Adjusted Reimbursement for People with Disabilities: A Diagnostic Approach Proposed for Missouri.* Boston: Medicaid Working Group, November 1995.
3. Alpha Center. The California Managed Risk Medical Insurance Board's Health Risk Adjusters Project. *Health Care Financing and Organization News and Progress,* November 1995.
4. Fowler E and Anderson G. Capitation adjustment for pediatric populations. *Pediatrics.* July 1996; Vol. 98 No.1:10–17.
5. Fox HB, McManus MA. *Medicaid Managed Care for Children with Chronic or Disabling Conditions: Improved Strategies for States and Plans.* Washington, DC: Fox Health Policy Consultants; 1996
6. American Academy of Pediatrics, Committee on Child Health Financing. Berman S, Gross R, Lewak N, eds. *A Pediatrician's Guide to Managed Care.* Elk Grove Village, IL: AAP; 1995. The resource guide is available from the AAP Division of Marketing and Publications, 141 Northwest Point Blvd, Elk Grove Village, IL 60007, 800/433-9016.

# CARE COORDINATION

## Problem Statement

Coordinating the care of certain children who either have or are at risk of having chronic conditions can be difficult, time-consuming, and costly. It also can be enjoyable and rewarding clinically. It can include some or all of the following functions:

- appointment scheduling and tracking
- family-focused psychosocial assessment
- outreach
- care planning and implementation
- assurance of access to care, authorization of services, service monitoring, and brokering
- resource management
- quality assurance
- public program eligibility determination
- linkages with schools and other community-based agencies and family support groups

Care coordination, however, can be complicated by the fact that many entities, in addition to the child's pediatrician and managed care plan, may have some responsibility for case management.

Four groups of children and their families often require care coordination services. They are as follows: (1) children using multiple health, mental health, early intervention, special education, or social services; (2) children whose families are experiencing significant difficulties, such as substance abuse, mental illness, or serious illness, which impair their ability to parent; (3) families without basic resources (eg, transportation, housing), where the lack of these resources interferes with their ability to access services; and (4) adolescents engaging in risk-taking behaviors (eg, substance abuse, early and unsafe sex, gang activity). Without an efficient, proactive system of care coordination or case management for these children and their families, adverse health and functional outcomes are predictable.

The following set of issues highlights the key areas of concern pediatricians encounter in providing care coordination. As a member of the care coordination team, pediatricians should be familiar with the issues and how they may affect the care planning process.

## Key Issues

- The identification of children and families who require care coordination services is highly variable. This is limited by the lack of a clear-cut definition of children with special health care needs. It is also limited by the fact that many managed care plans provide care coordination only to those requiring the highest cost care.

- There is a lack of consensus about terms, definitions, and standards for care coordination.

- Reimbursement to perform care coordination functions is seldom available or adequate. There are CPT codes that can be used for case management services and care planning oversight if recognized by payers.

- Many children only have access to medical case management in managed care plans, not comprehensive case management that includes coordinating health, education, and other related services. Medical case management is often aimed at cost management, with less attention to service coordination. It often does not have a preventive focus. Increasingly, managed care plans are developing disease-specific case management systems. Disease management programs organize care for a specific high-cost, high-volume diagnosis (eg, asthma, diabetes) with the intention of improving outcomes and lowering overall costs. Some pharmaceutical manufacturers have also created disease management programs that stress coordination of therapies.

- Families also play a central role in care coordination; however, their role is not often fully realized.

- Care coordination is often performed by multiple groups, including the primary care provider or, in some cases, the pediatric medical subspecialist, the managed care plan or insurer, the Title V Program for Children With Special Health Care Needs, and various other public programs. These programs may not coordinate with each other or staff involved may not understand the specific demands of simplifying the care coordination process. The result is an increased burden on providers for documentation and increased confusion of families about who, if anyone other than themselves, is responsible for specific aspects of the care.

- Most providers, plans, and state agencies have inadequate automation systems to support comprehensive care coordination.

## Summary of Approaches for Care Coordination for Children With Special Needs

1. ACCESS-MCH, assists state Title V Programs for Children With Special Health Care Needs in automating their case management systems for children with special health care needs. ACCESS-MCH maintains resources, documents best practices, and disseminates information on care coordination and automation. (ACCESS-MCH, Center for Automation and Care Coordination Enhancing Service Systems in Maternal and Child Health, 4634 Hollywood Blvd, Los Angeles, CA, 213/913-4400. In Massachusetts, ACCESS-MCH is located at Sweet Hall, Tufts University, Medford, MA 02155, 617/627-3626.)

2. Several case management software packages exist for children. For example, Automated Case Management Systems, Inc, in California has a generic care management system, Case Watch, which automates client registration, psychosocial assessment, progress note entry, service planning, resource matching, and reporting. It also has specific systems tailored to AIDS, early intervention, and homeless youth. (ACMS, Inc at 3301 Barham Blvd, No. 202, Los Angeles, CA 90068. 213/876-2273. Fax: 213/876-2033.)

Peter Martin Associates of Chicago, IL, offers several case management software products. Chicago's La Rabida Children's Hospital and Research Center adapted their prototype into the Family Care Tracking System (FACTS) to track referrals, intake, individualized service plans, and the involvement of community-based resources. (For information, contact Edward Hamlin, 2547 W Leland Ave, Chicago, IL 60625, 312/478-2400.)

3. Linkages and Outcomes for Children, based in the state of Washington, will assist managed care plans, public health agencies, social services, and schools in creating and using a uniform case management database to coordinate care across settings. (For information contact Donna Borgford-Parnell, Washington State Department of Health, PO Box 47880, Olympia, WA 98504-4850, 206/296-7412.)

## Implications for Practicing Pediatricians

There are several key principles to guide the development of improved care coordination services.

- The child's medical home should serve as a primary coordinator of medical care and should be aware of other case managers, health care professionals, and non-health care professionals involved with the child's care and coordinate the plan of care.[1] Depending on the specifics of who is involved on a particular child's team, the physician may or may not be the best lead person.

- Pediatricians should support families who ultimately have the main responsibility for care coordination within the plan.

- Distinctions between benefits management and service coordination should be clarified so that both goals can be achieved.

- The roles and qualifications of care coordinators should be specified at the outset to avoid duplication of efforts and inappropriate decision making. It may be wise to establish a series of meetings or conferences to clarify the roles, to identify potential problems up front, and to support the activities of the team.

- Adequate compensation and support for participation in care coordination should be offered. Always document the time spent on care coordination. This information can be used to demonstrate the need for higher compensation and illustrate the essential role played by the pediatrician. Also, find out whether the plan reimburses for the CPT codes for care plan oversight, case management services, and telephone calls.

- Pediatricians and families should try to be aware of other health care and social services that exist in the schools, community, and state. Pediatricians may want to obtain existing resource lists of the many services available in the community to share with the family. Many agencies develop these types of lists.

1. American Academy of Pediatrics, Ad Hoc Task Force on Definition of the Medical Home. The medical home. *Pediatrics.* 1992;90:774

# QUALITY OF CARE

## Problem Statement

Few quality-of-care measures exist to evaluate care of children with chronic conditions. One reason for this is that many chronic conditions affecting children are rare and few managed care plans have sufficient numbers of such children to collect statistically reliable information. Another reason is that there is a mistaken perception that very few children have chronic conditions. Finally, relatively little research has been conducted on pediatric quality of care. Because of the dearth of performance measures, payers, managed care organizations, pediatric providers, and families are at a disadvantage in evaluating and continuously improving quality of care for high-risk pediatric populations.

The following set of issues highlights the key areas of concern pediatricians encounter in evaluating the quality-of-care measures used and the protocols employed by managed care plans.

## Key Issues

- Quality-of-care measures used to evaluate pediatric clinical performance focus almost exclusively on primary and preventive care, using process not outcome measures. Beyond asthma, few process or outcome measures exist to evaluate clinical performance for children with chronic conditions, particularly those with rare conditions, developmental delays and disabilities, and behavioral and emotional conditions. Reliable and valid methods for severity adjustment are also lacking.

- Quality-of-care measures used to evaluate children's utilization of health services generally focus on preventive care (eg, EPSDT and immunizations), ambulatory care, emergency room services, inpatient hospital care, mental health and substance abuse services, and prescription drug use. The

ability to monitor utilization of special services such as ancillary therapy services, home health care, durable medical equipment, and medical supplies is critical for chronically ill children. Also, the inability to distinguish utilization of primary and specialty physician services in many administration data sets continues to be problematic.

- Quality-of-care measures used to evaluate children's access to care focus almost exclusively on the availability of primary care providers and waiting times for routine, urgent, and emergent care appointments. Measures such as the availability of linguistically appropriate providers are also being used. Few measures exist that address the unique access barriers and follow-up requirements for families whose children have chronic conditions (eg, special transportation services, times of clinic availability, easily accessible telephone advice, and follow-up systems). Also, when measuring access payers and plans seldom have documentation that relates to the availability of pediatric medical subspecialists, pediatric surgical specialists, mental health professionals with pediatric expertise, ancillary therapists with pediatric expertise, or hospitals specializing in the care of children.

- Quality-of-care measures used to evaluate member satisfaction focus primarily on adult satisfaction with care. Questions for children tend to be very broad — satisfaction with pediatric care overall, provider interest in pediatric patient, and pediatric medical care and treatment. Few member satisfaction survey instruments have been tested for Medicaid populations.

- Health plan management measures typically used include information on the plan's provider network — specifically, physician board certification and residency completion and the availability of primary care physicians, specialists, and mental health professionals. Clinical and care management systems, such as special quality and service improvement studies, utilization management techniques, new member orientation, and health education programs are also included. Seldom is this plan information specific to children.

There is evidence of quality-of-care measure used to gauge a plan's performance as it relates to pediatric care. A few examples of these measures are provided in the following section.

## Summary of Approaches for Quality of Care for Children With Special Health Care Needs

1. The National Committee on Quality Assurance (NCQA) released the first Medicaid HEDIS (Health Plan and Employer Data Information Set) in December 1995.[1] It is intended to assist state Medicaid agencies in producing performance measures specifically targeted to meet the needs of low-income women and children. A limitation of the HEDIS is that few measures exist for children with chronic conditions. The HEDIS also is not mandatory — states may choose to implement some or all of Medicaid HEDIS measures. Medicaid HEDIS is an adaptation of NCQA's HEDIS 2.0/2.5.[2] HEDIS 3.0, released January 1997, is an integrated measurement set that addresses a broader population, including Medicaid and Medicare recipients as well as privately insured persons and acute and chronic care. The measures used in HEDIS 3.0 closely resemble the Medicaid HEDIS measures.

The NCQA also completed a Report Card Pilot Project in collaboration with 21 health plans and key employer, consumer, health policy, and labor representatives.[3] The purpose of this project was to test the feasibility of implementing standardized performance measures. The measures were adapted from HEDIS 2.0 and, for children, include immunizations, low birth weight rates, asthma admission rates, and hospital days. The NCQA is also establishing an electronic database on health plan quality. The database will contain indicators of quality of care, accreditation status, and consumer satisfaction for health maintenance organizations. Employers, purchasing coalitions, benefits consulting organizations, consumers, health services researchers, and managed care plans will be able to access the database.

Recognizing the dearth of chronic care measures, NCQA has a chronic care project underway to develop measures for the management of chronic conditions: major depression, diabetes, coronary artery disease, and asthma. However, only the asthma measured is specifically designed for children ages 5 through 18. A model of care will be defined for those with mild, moderate, or severe asthma. Measures will address the health status of the population, compliance with treatment guidelines, episode prevention (examined by emergency room visits), episode characteristics (examined through the number of hospital days), and parent and/or patient satisfaction.

2. The Health Care Financing Administration (HCFA) has supported several projects as part of their Quality Assurance Reform Initiative (QARI).[4] Designed to improve the consistency of the oversight of Medicaid managed care quality across states and to assist states in updating and strengthening their quality assurance systems, QARI calls for HCFA to provide national standards, state guidance, and oversight. State Medicaid agencies are to monitor managed care plans, establish state standards, contract for external review, and define areas of study and joint planning with managed care organizations. External review organizations provide independent assessments of quality. Managed care organizations implement internal quality assurance requirements. Three states have been testing the QARI system for 2 years — Minnesota, Ohio, and Washington. The HCFA also produced a best-practice technical assistance guide for states to use in developing Health Care Quality Improvement Systems (HCQIS) for Medicaid managed care, which was produced in 1993.[5] A new revision of QARI is currently underway.

A series of HCFA-funded studies looking at the quality of Medicaid managed care are described below:

*Mathematica Policy Research* and *The Urban Institute* have been conducting an evaluation of five health reform demonstrations in Hawaii, Oklahoma, Rhode Island, Tennessee, and Vermont. The evaluation will address program organization and implementation, specifically new eligibility and premium-sharing arrangements, development and management of managed care organizations, and consumer and health provider reaction. Participants' access to, use of, and satisfaction with health services; the effects on program costs and expenditures; and the impact on persons with disabilities will also be studied.

*RAND* is developing and testing a clinically based method for assessing the quality of care delivered to women and children in managed care plans. Data will be analyzed based on quality scores across types of services (preventive, diagnostic, and treatment), type of condition (acute vs chronic), age group, socioeconomic group (Medicaid vs non-Medicaid), race and ethnicity, and length of time in plan.

3. The Agency for Health Care Policy and Research (AHCPR) has developed clinical practice guidelines for sickle cell disease, acute pain management for children and adolescents, early HIV infection, and otitis media with effusion. With the Maternal and Child Health Bureau and several other federal agencies and private foundations, AHCPR sponsored a conference to set an agenda for pediatric quality-of-care research in the spring of 1997. The AHCPR released a computer tool to make it easier for health plans, providers, and purchasers to choose and use clinical performance measures to assess the quality of the services they provide and purchase. CONQUEST 1.0, the Computerized Need-Created Quality Measurement Evaluation System (CONQUEST) summarizes information on approximately 1,200 clinical performance measures developed by public and private sector organizations to examine the quality of clinical care. It includes preprogrammed reports on measures and conditions and also allows users to perform tailored searches and create customized reports. [Contact the AHCPR Clearinghouse (800/358-9295) for CONQUEST 1.0 Materials (Publication No. 96-N009) or send a postcard to AHCPR Publications Clearinghouse, (Attn.: Publication No. 96-N009), PO Box 8547, Silver Spring, MD 20907.]

4. The Maternal and Child Health Bureau currently funds projects related to pediatric quality of care and managed care. They include:

   • New England SERVE, based in Boston, has developed indicators of quality and satisfaction for children with special health care needs served by managed care organizations.

• The state of Washington's Department of Health is developing and evaluating community-generated methods for monitoring health status and outcomes for special-needs children who are enrolled in the state's capitated arrangements. Outcomes monitored will include the child's functional health status, health and community services received, and family satisfaction with the health system.

• Oregon's Child Development and Rehabilitation Center has developed practice guidelines for use by the state Medicaid agency and participating managed care plans for children with cerebral palsy, spina bifida, and cleft lip and palate. Developed by a panel of pediatric experts, these guidelines include treatment goals, composition of the health care team, content of the initial evaluation and reevaluations, and frequency of visits. Guidelines for cystic fibrosis, Down syndrome, newborn screens, and asthma are currently under development.

• The Boston-based Research Consortium on Chronic Illness in Childhood is examining quality-of-care issues for children with special health care needs in managed care.

5. The American Academy of Pediatrics (AAP) has several activities underway related to quality of care. The Ambulatory Care Quality Improvement Program (ACQIP) assists physicians in evaluating their practices by comparing themselves to peers. Three aspects of practice are addressed: practice management, clinical management, and patient satisfaction. Participating practices are able to compare their results on the quality improvement exercises to national scores and to AAP recommended practices. To date, the following areas have been examined: hyperbilirubinemia in the healthy term newborn, monitoring otitis media, patient satisfaction with ear infection management, parents' perception of vision and hearing screening, vaccine storage, immunization medical record keeping, vaccine administration, patient satisfaction and immunizations, telephone advice, developmental assessments and medical record keeping, office management of

acute exacerbations of asthma in children, and patient satisfaction with asthma management. [Contact the American Academy of Pediatrics, Division of Quality Care, 141 Northwest Point Blvd, Elk Grove Village, IL 60007 (800/433-9016) for information on the ACQIP program.]

Another quality improvement resource is the AAP practice parameters. The practice parameters provide pediatricians with strategies and educational tools for patient management and clinical decision making. To date, practice parameters have been published on asthma, hyperbilirubinemia, otitis media, acute gastroenteritis, and neurodiagnosis of the child with a first simple febrile seizure.

Finally, the Academy's functional outcomes project is a program to develop quality-of-life measures for children with chronic conditions that are condition-specific and health-related. The long-range goal of the project is to develop multiple measures for several of the most common and/or severe conditions affecting children.

6. The National Association of Children's Hospitals and Related Institutions (NACHRI) released a report titled *Pediatric Excellence in Delivery Systems*, which includes criteria and measures for development of high-quality primary, acute, and chronic levels of care for children.

## Implications for Practicing Pediatricians

There are several issues that pediatricians may want to consider in order to strengthen pediatric quality-of-care measurement for this vulnerable population. Pediatricians should work with their state chapter and other child advocacy organizations in pediatric quality-of-care measurements for children with chronic conditions.

- Obtain from each managed care plan and state Medicaid office the information on the type of quality measures used to monitor performance for children generally and also for children with special needs. If Medicaid HEDIS is used, there will be insufficient attention to assess key performance in serving special-needs children. Suggest additional approaches to managed care plans, such as grouping many rare chronic conditions together and assessing plan performance related to early identification, provider capacity, and organization (including the use of multidisciplinary teams), specialty referrals, service utilization, care coordination, and/or family satisfaction.

- In addition to assessing in-plan performance, consider examining the extent to which children are accessing wraparound services or out-of-contract services provided by early intervention and special education programs as well as community-based and family support services. This is particularly important among privately insured children who may have limited coverage for chronic care services. For Medicaid-insured children, it is important since many states continue to finance many services outside of the capitated plan arrangement. Monitoring reasons for disen-rollment may also prove instructive.

- Encourage plans to expand the consumer satisfaction surveys of families whose children have chronic conditions. Family Voices and New England SERVE have developed tools that can be used to assess plan performance. (Contact Family Voices at The Federation for Children With Special Needs, 95 Berkeley St, Suite 104, Boston, MA 02116.) Encourage families to participate in both survey design and analysis and maintain a strong role in overall quality improvement programs.

- Recommend that children with special health care needs have annual assessments of health and functional status to monitor changes and relate them to the care plan. Either the QuICCC Instrument or the Child Health Questionnaire, described under the issue brief on identifying and defining children who have special health care needs, may be used for this purpose.

1. National Committee on Quality Assurance. *Medicaid HEDIS.* Washington, DC: National Committee on Quality Assurance; 1995

2. National Committee for Quality Assurance. *The Health Plan Employer Data and Information Set (HEDIS 2.0/2.5).* Washington, DC: NCQA; 1995

3. National Committee for Quality Assurance. *NCQA Report Card Plan Project/Technical Report.* Washington, DC: NCQA; 1994

4. Gold M, Felt S. Reconciling practice and theory: challenges in monitoring Medicaid managed-care quality. *Health Care Financing Rev.* 1995; 16: (4)

5. US Department of Health and Human Services. *A Health Care Quality Improvement System for Medicaid Managed Care: A Guide for States.* Washington, DC: HCQA; 1993

6. National Association of Children's Hospitals and Related Institutions. *Pediatric Excellence in Health Delivery Systems.* Alexandria, VA: National Association of Children's Hospitals and Related Institutions, 1996

# INTEGRATED SYSTEM DESIGN

## Problem Statement

No operational models exist of integrated pediatric managed care systems that incorporate personal medical care services, including behavioral health services, community health services, health-related early intervention and special education services, and other social and family support services. A few, however, are in the planning stages and are designed to serve a very small segment of the special-needs child population. For adults, two comprehensive demonstration programs are operational in a small but growing number of sites — social health maintenance organizations (SHMOs) and programs for all-inclusive care for the elderly (PACE). SHMOs have been designed to offer more long-term care benefits by pooling Medicare and other outside funds and to coordinate acute, long-term care, and other support services.[1] PACE integrates Medicare and Medicaid funds to provide a comprehensive array of acute and long-term care services.[2]

The American Academy of Pediatrics (AAP) and the National Association of Children's Hospitals and Related Institutions (NACHRI) released a statement on integrated child health care networks in 1994.[3] They recommended that such a network would be:

- expert in meeting the full continuum of children's preventive, primary, acute, subspecialty, post-acute, habilitative and rehabilitative, and long-term care, as well as mental health care needs;

- organized to work together to assume responsibility for managing the full continuum of care for a specific population of children; and to provide quality care in a cost-efficient manner; and

- accountable to the public for the health status — the "wellness" — of the population of children covered, as well as their use of services, according to agreed-upon measures of children's health status and pediatric care outcomes.

In many areas, children's hospitals in partnership with community pediatricians are forming capitated pediatric products for all children as well as for special-needs children. These pediatric networks are contracting primarily with managed care organizations to provide preventive, primary, and chronic medical care services. Another pediatric managed care innovation that has received a great deal of attention is the Washington, DC, program called Health Services for Children With Special Health Care Needs (described on the following page). Still, these pediatric managed care initiatives have only begun to explore the full potential of integrated services for children.

The following set of issues highlights the key areas of concern pediatricians may encounter in developing integrated systems of care.

## Key Issues

- There has been little investment in demonstrations and evaluations to develop integrated pediatric managed care models.

- Few purchasers appear to be interested in buying a children's product, preferring instead to contract with managed care plans that can serve entire families.

- Without adequate risk adjustment or risk-sharing arrangements and pooling of funds from multiple sources, plans that offer such comprehensive service are likely to attract a disproportionate share of children with chronic or disabling conditions.

- Complex federal and state rules and requirements for existing categorical programs serving children can limit the feasibility of combining funding and services from various sources.

## Summary of Integrated System Designs for Children With Special Health Care Needs

A few models do exist that integrate the various health care services chronically ill children require into one network. The systems described below appear to be the most comprehensive to date.

- Health Services for Children With Special Needs, Inc. (HSCSN) in Washington, DC, was granted a Medicaid Section 1115 Demonstration Waiver to provide comprehensive services to SSI-eligible children. Approximately 3,200 children will be offered the option to enroll in HSCSN or to remain in the fee-for-service system. HSCSN provides services currently available under Medicaid and, in addition, comprehensive care management, transportation and telephones, and family support.

- Ohio is a demonstration site for a managed care program for disabled recipients and recipients who are chronically ill receiving Medicaid. Their project, Accessing Better Care (ABC), requires providers to offer a flexible benefit package that includes home and community-based care and case management to assure coordination of all facets of patient care. Individuals with disabilities are to be included in the program design. Two bidders were selected to enroll patients as of January 1995. The Ohio State University Medical Center and the Nationwide Insurance HMO, InHealth, have partnered to provide a full array of medical services and out-patient specialty clinics, case management teams, and a network of community-based medical and social service providers. Columbus Children's Hospital has contracted through Ohio State University to provide all pediatric services. MetroHealth System and United Health Care have partnered to provide services as the other bidder.

## Implications for Practicing Pediatricians

Despite the AAP and NACHRI's support for integrated pediatric system designs in capitated managed care plans, relatively few innovations have occurred in this area. There are, however, several steps that pediatricians may pursue to promote greater service integration.

- Collaborate with managed care plans in using new improved screening tools to assess child and family risks and in developing community-based health education and family support services. Information obtained from the screening tools can be used to develop an inventory of services chronically ill children may need. This is a starting point in identifying the core components of an integrated system of care.

- Work to strengthen and broaden care coordination between managed care plans and community-based health and related services that are provided out-of-plan. Encourage the formation of ad hoc teams to identify ways to strengthen care coordination. A strong and effective care coordination process not only benefits the patient and family but also can conserve resource by avoiding duplication of effort.

- Encourage managed care plans to meet with publicly funded programs to determine the potential of joint funding, shared staffing arrangements, and collaborative program planning and evaluation.

1. Manton KG, Newcomer RJ, Lowrimore GR, et al. Social/health maintenance organization and fee-for-service health outcomes over time. *Health Care Financing Rev.* 1993;15(2):173–202
2. Kane RL, Illston LH, Miller NA. Quantitative analysis of the Program of All-Inclusive Care for the Elderly (PACE). *The Gerontologist.* 1992;32(6):771–780
3. Integrated Child Health Care Networks. Statement by the American Academy of Pediatrics (AAP) and the National Association of Children's Hospital and Related Institutions (NACHRI). 1994

# POLICY
# STATEMENTS

# AMERICAN ACADEMY OF PEDIATRICS

## The Medical Home (RE9262)

Ad Hoc Task Force on Definition of the Medical Home

The American Academy of Pediatrics believes that the medical care of infants, children, and adolescents ideally should be accessible, continuous, comprehensive, family centered, coordinated, and compassionate. It should be delivered or directed by well-trained physicians who are able to manage or facilitate essentially all aspects of pediatric care. The physician should be known to the child and family and should be able to develop a relationship of mutual responsibility and trust with them. These characteristics define the "medical home" and describe the care that has traditionally been provided by pediatricians in an office setting. In contrast, care provided through emergency departments, walk-in clinics, and other urgent-care facilities is often less effective and more costly.

We should strive to attain a "medical home" for all of our children. Although geographic barriers, personnel constraints, practice patterns, and economic and social forces make the ideal "medical home" unobtainable for many children, we believe that comprehensive health care of infants, children, and adolescents, wherever delivered, should encompass the following services:

1. Provision of preventive care including, but not restricted to, immunizations, growth and development assessments, appropriate screening, health care supervision, and patient and parental counseling about health and psychosocial issues.
2. Assurance of ambulatory and inpatient care for acute illnesses, 24 hours a day, 7 days a week; during the working day, after hours, on weekends, 52 weeks of the year.
3. Provision of care over an extended period of time to enhance continuity.
4. Identification of the need for subspecialty consultation and referrals and knowing from whom and where these can be obtained. Provision of medical information about the patient to the consultant. Evaluation of the consultant's recommendations, implementation of recommendations that are indicated and appropriate, and interpretation of these to the family.
5. Interaction with school and community agencies to be certain that special health needs of the individual child are addressed.
6. Maintenance of a central record and data base containing all pertinent medical information about the child, including information about hospitalizations. This record should be accessible, but confidentiality must be assured.

Medical care of infants, children, and adolescents must sometimes be provided in locations other than physician's offices. However, unless these locations provide all of the services listed above, they do not meet the definition of a medical home. Other venues for children's care include hospital outpatient clinics, school-based and school-linked clinics, community health centers, health department clinics, and others. However, wherever given, medical care coverage must be constantly available. It should be supervised by physicians well-trained in primary pediatric medicine, preferably pediatricians. Whenever possible, the physician should be physically present where the care is provided; but it may be necessary for the physician to direct other health care providers such as nurses, nurse practitioners, and physician assistants off site. Whether physically present or not, the physician must act as the child's advocate and assume control and ultimate responsibility for the care that is provided.

Ad Hoc Task Force on Definition of the Medical Home
Michael D. Dickens, MD
John L. Green, MD
Alan E. Kohrt, MD
Howard A. Pearson, MD

PEDIATRICS (ISSN 0031 4005). Copyright © 1992 by the American Academy of Pediatrics.

# AMERICAN ACADEMY OF PEDIATRICS

## The Medical Home Statement Addendum: Pediatric Primary Health Care

(RE9262)

PRIMARY HEALTH CARE is described as accessible and affordable, first contact, continuous and comprehensive, and coordinated to meet the health needs of the individual and the family being served.

PEDIATRIC PRIMARY HEALTH CARE encompasses health supervision and anticipatory guidance; monitoring physical and psychosocial growth and development; age-appropriate screening; diagnosis and treatment of acute and chronic disorders; management of serious and life-threatening illness and, when appropriate, referral of more complex conditions; and provision of first contact care as well as coordinated management of health problems requiring multiple professional services. PEDIATRIC PRIMARY HEALTH CARE for children and adolescents is family oriented and incorporates community resources and strengths, needs and risk factors, and sociocultural sensitivities into strategies for care delivery and clinical practice. PEDIATRIC PRIMARY HEALTH CARE is best delivered within the context of a "medical home," where comprehensive, continuously accessible and affordable care is available and delivered or supervised by qualified child health specialists.

The PEDIATRICIAN, because of training (which includes four years of medical school education, plus an additional three or more years of intensive training devoted solely to all aspects of medical care for children and adolescents), coupled with the demonstrated interest in and total professional commitment to the health care of infants, children, adolescents and young adults, is the most appropriate provider of PEDIATRIC PRIMARY HEALTH CARE.

# AMERICAN ACADEMY OF PEDIATRICS

## The Pediatrician and the "New Morbidity" (RE9335)

Committee on Psychosocial Aspects of Child and Family Health

### THE CHALLENGE

A decade has passed since the American Academy of Pediatrics (AAP) defined the role of the pediatrician in providing increased attention to the prevention, early detection, and management of the various behavioral, developmental, and social functioning problems encountered in pediatric practice.[1] These problems, called the "new morbidity,"[2] are not really "new"; they have always affected children, but many have become more prevalent. For example, the number of children and adolescents with activity limitation caused by a chronic health condition with attendant psychological problems currently approaches 8%.[3] The number of children living with divorced mothers doubled between 1970 and 1986. The suicide rate for male adolescents has doubled since 1960.[4] Because of the prevalance of these problems, the peditrician is being asked to expand the traditional role of health supervision and management of physical illnesses to address psychosocial and behavioral problems more effectively.

### THE BARRIERS

To achieve this goal, pediatricians must overcome educational, economic, and time management obstacles, despite tremendous strides in the development of an educational blueprint,[5] an ever-increasing knowledge base, and a growing cadre of educators.[6] Pediatric residency training is focused on major physical illness in tertiary care hospitals and to a limited degree on behavioral issues. Training in ambulatory settings has expanded, although training in behavioral pediatrics remains limited in many residency programs. In 1987, the Residency Review Committee added a requirement for behavioral teaching, although the specific time requirement for training in behavioral pediatrics is undefined. Consequently many pediatricians have completed training with limited instruction in psychosocial issues. Expanding developmental, behavioral, and adolescent training during residency would better equip the pediatrician to address these new morbidities.

Better education of pediatricians is necessary but not sufficient to address the new morbidity. Many children with pressing needs never reach the pediatrician or other child care professionals because of barriers to health care access. In practice, even the pediatrician with a well-rounded education experiences time constraints and inadequate reimbursement for the effort required to address behavioral problems.

There are additional barriers to addressing behavioral problems. Current systems for classifying mental disorders in children do not adequately describe the types of psychosocial and behavioral problems encountered by pediatricians. Another concern is the increasing reliance on a pathology-based model for screening mental health problems. Although behavioral checklists help screen children with psychiatric problems needing referral,[8] the pediatrician's potential area of competence is greater than mere screening for major mental disorders.

### REALISTIC OBJECTIVES

The pediatrician's professional competence and job satisfaction in handling behavioral issues can be enhanced by several changes.

#### Clarify the Expanded Areas of Pediatric Competence

Pediatricians need the following areas of knowledge:

1. Physical and environmental factors affecting behavior, including risk factors, their impact, prevention, and management;
2. Normal variations of development and behavior, and how to help parents deal with them;
3. Behavior affecting physical health, including risk factors (eg, medical noncompliance, smoking), their impact, prevention, and management;
4. Mild and moderate behavioral problems, including detection, evaluation, and management;
5. Severe behavioral deviations, including recognition, preliminary evaluation, and appropriate referral.

#### Develop Interviewing Skills

Pediatricians depend heavily on interviewing skills in their evaluation of patients. Interviewing skills are an important diagnostic and therapeutic method for managing behavioral issues. The interviewing and evaluation process sorts through the complex data presented by parents and other caretakers, arrives at an assessment of the status of the child and family, assesses what is needed to alter significant family interactions to benefit the child, and determines appropriate referral.

#### Establish a Comprehensive Mental Health Model

A mental health model that adequately integrates physical and mental issues should be developed for

This statement has been approved by the Council on Child and Adolescent Health.

The recommendations in this policy statement do not indicate an exclusive course of treatment or serve as a standard of medical care. Variations, taking into account individual circumstances, may be appropriate.

primary care. A comprehensive model integrating those issues and considering aspects of adjustment and adaptation among children and families is needed. The AAP Task Force on Coding for Mental Health in Children is developing a Diagnostic and Statistical Manual for Primary Care (DSM-PC). A nosology in primary care is being developed that incorporates a developmental perspective and categorizes normal variation and problems as well as mental health disorders.[9]

The current psychiatric diagnostic terminology (*Diagnostic and Statistical Manual of Mental Disorders*, 3rd edition revised, and *International Classification of Diseases*, 9th revision), is useful to child psychiatrists and other mental health professionals, but it is not designed to meet the needs of the pediatrician. The terminology and model do not provide a meaningful framework for organizing the information gathered by a skillful pediatric interviewer. A comprehensive mental health model that is appropriate for the pediatric setting, considers positive as well as negative aspects of adjustment, and encourages the clinician to make the behavioral diagnostic judgments is needed.

### Improve Pediatric Counseling Skills

Counseling is a skill possessed by pediatricians but underutilized in the management of behavioral problems.[10] With a combination of knowledge, interviewing skills, and diagnostic understanding, pediatricians can effectively counsel patients and families and improve most behavioral problems they encounter. Many pediatricians may need to improve their performance in these areas in order to utilize their skills more effectively. For example, pediatricians can allay parents' fears and provide reassurance by bringing information about the wide range of normal behavior to the clinical encounter.[11] Pediatricians may underestimate the therapeutic value of the interview itself, a value that is gained before any counseling is done.

### Allocate Time Realistically

Child health supervision visits are effective for detecting physical abnormalities and preventing illness. When psychosocial issues are detected during such a visit, there may be insufficient time to address the problems adequately. Developmental issues reflecting normal variations may be managed within the context of a health supervision visit. More complex situations, such as divorce, bereavement, or school failure, require additional visits with ample time to discuss the problem. The individual skill level of the pediatrician will determine the complexity of psychosocial issues that can be managed effectively.

### Improve Referral Skills

Some children have complex psychosocial problems that need referral. Some children may be better served in an alternate setting, such as a school or community mental health center, where a wider range of resources is available for the child and family.[12]

The child's environment, such as a stressful marital separation, can pose a threat to a child even though he or she may not yet manifest any ill effects. Pediatricians with appropriate clinical knowledge, interviewing, and counseling skills are more likely to make timely and effective referrals.

The pediatrician's relationship with the school system and knowledge of the available social and mental health referral sources affects referral. Pediatricians must be familiar with mental health professionals who can manage complex problems identified in a typical pediatric practice.

### Revise Allocation of Resources

Resources are needed to address psychosocial morbidity and to compensate for past inattention to these problems. The quantity and quality of resident training in this area must be improved to allow for acquisition of requisite knowledge and skills. Reimbursement for the management of children with psychosocial problems must be revised to allow pediatricians the additional time required to perform this vital role.

### CONCLUSION

Implementing these objectives would make the pediatrician more effective in managing the "new morbidity." The cooperation of pediatric training program directors, educators, and practicing pediatricians is required. As new "epidemics" such as violence, poverty, technology-dependent children, drug-addicted infants, and human immunodeficiency virus continue to emerge, pediatric and pediatric-related organizations will need to continuously expand a mental health model that encompasses a classification scheme and new training curricula. Such efforts will gain momentum as pediatricians experience the satisfaction of growing professional competence and the sense of achievement that comes with effectively managing children's psychosocial problems.

Committee on Psychosocial Aspects of Child and Family Health, 1993 to 1994
Martin T. Stein, MD, Chair
William B. Carey, MD
Stanford B. Friedman, MD
Michael S. Jellinek, MD
Lucy Osborn, MD
Ellen C. Perrin, MD
Deborah Tolchin, MD
Mark L. Wolraich, MD

Liaison Representative
Mervyn Fox, MD
Canadian Paediatric Society

Consultants
George J. Cohen, MD, National Consortium for Child Mental Health Services
Robert Pantell, MD, University of California-San Francisco

### REFERENCES

1. American Academy of Pediatrics, Committee on Psychosocial Aspects of Child Family Health. Pediatrics and the psychosocial aspects of child and family health. *Pediatrics*. 1982;70:126–127

2. Haggerty RJ, Roghmann KJ, Pless IB. *Child Health and the Community*. New York, NY: John Wiley Sons; 1975

3. Gortmaker SL, Sappenfield W. Chronic childhood disorders: prevalence and impact. *Pediatr Clin North Am*. 1984;31:3–18

4. *US Children and Their Families: Current Conditions and Recent Trends, 1989*. A report together with additional views of the Select Committee on Children, Youth, and Families. US House of Representatives. Washington, DC: US Government Printing Office; 1989

5. American Academy of Pediatrics, Task Force on Pediatric Education. *The Future of Pediatric Education*. Evanston, IL: American Academy of Pediatrics; 1978

6. Martini CJ. Graduate medical education in the changing environment of medicine. *JAMA*. 1992;268:1097–1105

7. Dworkin PH. British and American recommendations for developmental monitoring: the role of surveillance. *Pediatrics*. 1989;84:1000–1010

8. Jellinek MS, Murphy JM. Screening for psychosocial disorders in pediatric practice. *AJDC*. 1988;142:1153–1157

9. Fleischman D. Experts to develop 'landmark' mental health coding. *AAP News*. December 1991;7:1,17

10. Costello EJ. Primary care pediatrics and child psychopathology: a review of diagnostic, treatment, and referral practice. *Pediatrics*. 1986;78:1044–1051

11. Casey PH, Whitt JK. Effect of the pediatrician on the mother-infant relationship. *Pediatrics*. 1980;65:815–820

12. American Academy of Pediatrics, Ad Hoc Task Force on Definition of the Medical Home. The medical home. *Pediatrics*. 1992;90:774

# AMERICAN ACADEMY OF PEDIATRICS

## Guiding Principles for Managed Care Arrangements for the Health Care of Infants, Children, Adolescents, and Young Adults

Committee on Child Health Financing                    (RE9519)

Faced with unprecedented growth in health care costs, employers, state Medicaid programs, and other purchasers of care have turned from traditional fee-for-service reimbursement to managed care plans in an attempt to find the most efficient strategies that provide access to quality health care while controlling costs. During this period of change in the delivery and financing of health care services, new and expanded efforts are needed to strengthen managed care systems serving infants, children, adolescents and young adults (hereinafter referred to collectively as "children") and their families.

The American Academy of Pediatrics (AAP) urges caution in designing and implementing managed care for children for several reasons—disruptions in provider-patient relationships; barriers to appropriate pediatric referrals and delays in treatment authorization[1]; limited quality-of-care measures appropriate for children[2]; lack of pediatric risk adjustment payment mechanisms[3]; limited coordination with public health, education, and social services systems[4]; and a general paucity of research on children in managed care.[5] Concern also has been raised about the adverse effects of shifting resources from providing medical services to generating excessive profit in for-profit health care plans. Many of the same criticisms can be made of traditional fee-for-service plans as well.

Managed care plans typically employ certain cost and utilization management features. (A glossary of managed care terminology is in the AAP publication *A Pediatrician's Guide to Managed Care.*[6]) It is important to monitor the impact of cost-containment measures on the quality and outcome of medical services for children. The financial arrangements often include capitation, discounted charges and fee schedules, and performance incentives. The features of utilization management generally include precertification, concurrent review and discharge planning, "gatekeeping" or case management, preauthorization, physician practice profiling, and high-cost case management. These financial and utilization incentives and disincentives should be structured to preserve and, when appropriate, extend access to comprehensive and coordinated preventive, acute, and chronic care for all children.

By including the precepts of primary care in the delivery of services, managed care can be a tool to increase access to a full range of health care providers and services. On the other hand, managed care can result in underutilization of appropriate services and reduced quality of care. Such underutilization could result from patient and physician disincentives to appropriate utilization and restrictions on access to pediatric specialty providers and tertiary care centers. Other access restrictions could block utilization of necessary related services such as mental health, social work services, developmental evaluation, occupational, physical, and speech and language therapies, school-linked clinics, and other public health service providers.

When a state has mandated participation in Medicaid managed care plans, it should implement rigorous regulatory oversight to ensure the quality and financial viability of participating managed care plans. In addition, in states where enrollment in managed care plans is mandatory, Medicaid beneficiaries should have the freedom to choose among two or more managed health care plans and participating public and private providers.[7] In areas where only one managed care plan is available, particularly rural areas, families should be able to choose their individual physicians.[7]

The AAP seeks to work in partnership with families, other health and health-related professionals, federal and state governments, employers, and the managed care industry to implement the following principles of managed care for children. These principles—regarding access to primary and specialty pediatric services, treatment authorization, quality of care, and financing and reimbursement—are intended to maximize the positive potential of managed care and to minimize any negative impact on health care for children.

### PRINCIPLES OF MANAGED CARE FOR CHILDREN

#### Access to Appropriate Primary Care Providers

1. Choice of primary care providers for children must include pediatricians.
2. Primary care pediatricians should serve as the child's medical home[8] and assure the delivery of comprehensive preventive, acute, and chronic care services. They should be accessible 24 hours a day, 7 days a week, or have appropriate coverage arrangements.
3. The role of the "gatekeeper" should be assumed by the primary care pediatrician (ie, the physician who assures that all referrals are medically necessary). This function might be transferred to a

pediatric specialist team for certain children with complex physical health problems (eg, those with special health care needs such as cystic fibrosis, juvenile rheumatoid arthritis, etc) if the specialist assumes both responsibility and financial risk for primary and specialty care. For certain physical, developmental, mental health, and social problems, the gatekeeper should seek the assistance of a multidisciplinary team with participation by appropriate public programs (eg, Title V Program for Children with Special Health Care Needs).

4. Families should receive education at the time of enrollment to understand fully how managed care arrangements work, including the need to obtain all health care services and referrals from the primary care provider. Incentives to reward families who comply with such plan guidelines should be explored.

### Access to Pediatric Specialty Services

1. When the services of a physician specialist or other health care professional are needed by children, plans should use providers with appropriate pediatric training and expertise. Pediatric-trained physician specialists, including pediatric medical and surgical specialists, should have completed an appropriate fellowship in their area of expertise and be certified by specialty boards in a timely fashion if certification is available. These practitioners should be engaged actively in the ongoing practice of their pediatric specialty and should participate in continuing medical education in this area.

2. There should be no financial barriers to access for pediatric specialty care above and beyond customary plan requirements for specialty care.

3. Plans should contract with the appropriate number and mix of geographically accessible pediatric-trained physician specialists and tertiary care centers for children.

4. Referral criteria for pediatric specialty providers should be developed. These criteria may include age of patient, specific diagnoses, severity of conditions, and logistical considerations (eg, geographical access and cultural competence).

5. An efficient process for approving referrals to pediatric specialists, in- and out-of-plan, should be developed and publicized widely to plan members.

### Treatment Authorization

1. Families and providers should be fully informed of the plan's participating providers. This should include an up-to-date listing of plan participants in which practices are currently open to patients insured by the managed care plan. Identification of primary care providers and required copayments should be listed on the patient's insurance card.

2. The treatment authorization process, which is initiated by the gatekeeper, should encourage and facilitate timely, appropriate referral for specialty consultations, hospital inpatient and outpatient care, and other treatments.

3. Plans should provide timely responses to treatment authorization requests, based on the nature and urgency of the patient's needs, including 24-hour access and approvals in the case of emergencies. Pediatricians should be leery of managed care contracts that require them to certify all emergency room visits.

4. Plans should provide a timely appeals process that includes direct discussions between the reviewing panel, the patient's pediatrician, the relevant specialists and, if appropriate, an internal review by an independent panel of pediatricians experienced in the treatment of the patient's illness.

### Quality Assurance

1. Health plan coverage policies (including limitations on the amount, duration, and scope of services; cost-sharing requirements; and participating providers) should be clear, simply written, and readily understood by all families.[9] Written standards should be established regarding access to primary care, referrals to specialty services, and protocols for service. Plans should also designate a special department from which potential enrollees can obtain information on the plan.

2. Pediatricians and pediatric specialists should play an active role in developing quality assurance mechanisms and ensuring quality of care in any cost-containment process.[9]

3. Plans should utilize quality-of-care measures for children, including assessments of structure, process, and health and functional outcomes (eg, compliance with pediatric preventive standards including, but not limited to, immunization rates and referrals for chronic physical and mental health problems).

4. Quality management should include appropriate peer review,[9] with pediatric cases reviewed by pediatricians.

5. Plans should create incentives to promote early identification of health problems among children.

6. States should publish uniform data that allow consumers and purchasers the opportunity to evaluate and compare performance including financial characteristics among competing plans.

### Financing and Reimbursement

1. Capitation rates should be developed that cover all the health care needs of children as defined by the AAP policy statement "Scope of Health Care Benefits for Infants, Children, and Adolescents Through Age 21 Years"[10] and the periodicity of visits in the Academy's "Recommendation for Preventive Pediatric Health Care."[11] Capitation rates for children should also take into account age, chronicity, and severity of underlying health problems and geographic considerations. No copayments should be applied to preventive services.

2. Medicaid managed care plans reimbursing physicians for pediatric care on a fee-for-service basis should set fees at a rate that is at least 90% of the

usual, customary, or reasonable (UCR) or equivalent to those in Medicare, whichever is higher[7].

3. If managed care plans use a resource-based relative value scale (RBRVS) as the basis for their fee schedule, they should adopt the pediatric work values currently under development through the American Medical Association/Specialty Society Relative Value Scale Update Committee (RUC).

4. Special financing arrangements should be made for financing medically necessary specialty services and case management for children to ensure that pediatric services are not undervalued in terms of practice, professional liability, and physician work values.

5. To ensure continuation of high-quality services for children, primary care physicians should be protected against undue financial risk. Risk levels for primary care office-based pediatricians should be on an aggregate, not an individual basis.

6. Federal requirements for capitalization should apply to all managed care plans. Federal and state governments should preapprove all contracts with managed care plans whose enrollees are primarily Medicaid-insured and require both the federal and state governments to guarantee provider payments if plans become insolvent.

## CONCLUSION

The AAP recommends that careful attention be devoted to the design, implementation, and evaluation of managed care plans serving children, including those with special health care needs. The AAP seeks to collaborate with managed care plans in adopting these guiding principles to assure access to high-quality pediatric services.

COMMITTEE ON CHILD HEALTH FINANCING, 1994 TO 1995
Stephen Berman, MD, Chair
Joseph C. Bogdan, MD
Gilbert A. Buchanan, MD
John S. Curran, MD
Arthur Garson, MD
Robert D. Gross, MBA, MD
Neal Halfon, MD, MPH
Norman Lewak, MD
Richard Nelson, MD

## REFERENCES

1. Cartland JDC, Yudkowsky BK. Barriers to pediatric referral in managed care systems. *Pediatrics*. 1992;89:183–192
2. Fox HB, McManus MA. *Medicaid Managed Care Arrangements and Their Impact on Children and Adolescents: A Briefing Report*. Washington, DC: Fox Health Policy Consultants; 1992
3. Anderson G. *Importance of Risk Adjusters to Children and Children's Hospitals*. Baltimore, MD: Center for Hospital Finance and Management, Johns Hopkins University; 1993
4. Fox HB, Wicks LB. *State Efforts to Maintain a Role for Publicly Funded Providers in a Medicaid Managed Care Environment*. Washington, DC: Fox Health Policy Consultants; 1993
5. Freund DA, Lewit EM. Managed care for children and pregnant women: promises and pitfalls. *Future Children*. Fall 1993:92–122
6. American Academy of Pediatrics, Committee on Child Health Financing. Berman S, Gross RD, Lewak N, eds. *A Pediatrician's Guide to Managed Care*. Elk Grove Village, IL: American Academy of Pediatrics; 1995
7. American Academy of Pediatrics, Committee on Child Health Financing. Medicaid policy statement. *Pediatrics*. 1994;93:135–136
8. American Academy of Pediatrics, Ad Hoc Task Force on Definition of the Medical Home. The medical home. *Pediatrics*. 1992;90:774
9. American Academy of Pediatrics, Committee on Child Health Financing. Principles of child health care financing. *Pediatrics*. 1993;91:506–507
10. American Academy of Pediatrics, Committee on Child Health Financing. Scope of health care benefits for infants, children, and adolescents through age 21 years. *Pediatrics*. 1993;91:508
11. American Academy of Pediatrics, Committee on Practice and Ambulatory Medicine. Recommendations for preventive pediatric health care. *AAP News*. July 1991;7:19

# AMERICAN ACADEMY OF PEDIATRICS

## Liability and Managed Care       (RE9638)

Committee on Medical Liability

**ABSTRACT.** This statement is intended to inform practitioners of the liability issues arising from managed care arrangements. Although it is not possible for pediatricians to completely insulate themselves from all liability in these areas, this statement offers a number of strategies to decrease the chances of being successfully sued. However, because case law within this realm is constantly evolving in each state, these serve only as guidelines and are subject to both local and emerging developments.

Although managed care has existed since the 1930s, it has only recently affected the majority of pediatricians. With managed care as a way of life for at least 80% of pediatricians,[1] a new set of medicolegal issues is emerging. In addition to this, a pediatrician now has to contend with a new set of financial as well as medical issues. The most common areas that affect pediatricians include utilization review, compensation through financial incentives, termination policies for both the physician and the patient, abandonment, and limitation on referrals and testing. Although pediatric care often involves parental, as opposed to patient, decision-making, for ease of reference in discussing these issues, the term "patient" is used throughout this statement. This term is used with the understanding that it refers to either the minor patient or the guardian(s), as appropriate and as consistent with the Academy's policy.

## UTILIZATION REVIEW

In the past, pediatricians made decisions about a patient's treatment based primarily on what the pediatrician perceived were the patient's medical needs and wishes. Due to the public's increased awareness of the high cost of medical care, its demand to curb those costs, and the fiscal methods used by managed care to meet these demands, the pediatrician can often be placed in a very uncomfortable and legally risky position.

The cornerstone of legal cases dealing with the issue of utilization review is *Wickline v State of California*.[2] The court in that case stated that the responsibility for deciding a patient's medical course belonged to the treating physician, not to the insurance company. It went on to say that those administering utilization review programs could be held liable if the programs were administered in an arbitrary or

negligent manner, and that the treating physician could not point to the health care payor as the liability "scapegoat." A more recent case, *Wilson v Blue Cross of Southern California*,[3] upheld portions of *Wickline* but greatly increased a health maintenance organization's liability in the area of utilization review, although it did not absolve the physician from liability for inappropriate or improper treatment.

As case law continues to evolve in this area, it is important for pediatricians who are subject to utilization review to consider the following:

*Plan Issues*
- Reviewers must include at least a registered nurse or physician, preferably a pediatrician.
- Any case in which approval was denied must be reviewed by a physician, preferably a pediatrician.
- There must be a reasonable appeals process in place.
- The physician reviewer must be available to discuss any denials over the phone.

If a contract does not contain the above-mentioned provisions, the pediatrician needs to renegotiate the contract with the managed care company.

*Pediatrician Issues*
- Pediatricians should use the entire appeals process to render the most appropriate care for their patients.
- Pediatricians should document all conversations regarding utilization review issues.
- In the rare case that a pediatrician cannot reach a reasonable agreement with utilization reviewers, the pediatrician should discuss with the patient the option of paying independently for medical care received outside of his or her insurance coverage. It is important to document this "informed refusal" if the patient chooses to refrain from receiving the noncovered care.

## INCENTIVE OR BONUS PROGRAMS

Although it has never been proved that incentive programs really do change physician behavior and decrease medical costs, they nonetheless continue to be used by managed care organizations. It is very difficult to defend one's position in cases in which there is direct financial gain attached to medical decision-making. Pediatricians considering involvement with a program that uses incentive or bonus plans should consider the following:

PEDIATRICS (ISSN 0031 4005). Copyright © 1996 by the American Academy of Pediatrics.

- In most cases, a broad-based program is easier to defend. These programs are based on the actions or expenditures of a group of physicians instead of one individual physician and on a time frame that considers the actions over a month, quarter, or year instead of each individual episode of care.
- A program that is tied not only to utilization but also to quality of care is far superior to a program that does not consider quality.

## TERMINATION

Another area of risk is that of termination of the contract. Any contract that a physician signs should clearly state both the company's and the physician's responsibility with regard to termination of the contract. The contract should list what events or actions can lead to termination by either party and the length of time necessary to terminate the contract.

The contract should also discuss issues surrounding termination of the physician/patient relationship. These include, but are not limited to, physician notification of patient termination and under what conditions a physician can terminate his or her relationship with a patient. Many managed care organizations have clauses in the contracts that allow termination of the physician-patient relationship in the event of a patient's continuous gross noncompliance with the treatment plan or a patient physically or verbally abusing the physician. In all cases, the events used to justify termination must be well-documented.

When a patient-physician relationship is to be terminated, it is important for appropriate, timely notification to occur so as not to constitute abandonment.

## ABANDONMENT

Although it may ultimately be the responsibility of the managed care company to notify patients that their primary care physician is no longer a provider within their organization, it is prudent for the pediatrician to notify the patient of a change of status within the organization. To best reduce the risk of an accusation of abandonment, at least 30 days before leaving, the physician should notify each patient affected by registered mail. Included in this letter may be a list of providers within the organization who are available to the patient.

Notification alone, however, may not be sufficient to avoid a claim of abandonment. If the care of the patient cannot be transferred expeditiously, the patient may continue to have a right to care despite the lack of a contract between the physician and the managed care organization. The physician similarly may be bound to provide treatment to a patient even in the event of the plan's financial insolvency.

## LIMITS ON TESTING AND REFERRALS

There are a variety of methods that managed care organizations use to limit referrals and testing. One method commonly used is the physician "report card." The company keeps track of the number and cost of testing and referrals ordered by each physician. The physician is then compared with his or her peers. These numbers can be very misleading depending on a variety of factors, such as patient age and severity of illness

within the physician's practice. The pressure that might be associated with this type of oversight may cause an individual physician to withhold necessary testing and/or referrals inappropriately.

Another way in which a managed care company may involve itself in the referral process is by limiting those specialists to whom a primary care provider can refer. It is important that a pediatrician be able to make referrals to pediatric medical subspecialists and pediatric surgeons. There is legal precedent for physician liability based on making referrals to a subspecialist that the pediatrician knew or should have known was inappropriate or incompetent. If a plan denies a referral to a pediatric medical subspecialist or pediatric surgeon, the pediatrician should notify the patient of the option of paying out-of-pocket for the consultation and, if necessary, obtain a written "informed refusal."

## HOLD HARMLESS CLAUSES

"Hold harmless" clauses are often found within managed care contracts. These clauses place the physician at total risk in the event of a medical malpractice suit and relieve the managed care organization of any liability. A pediatrician must attempt to negotiate with the managed care company to have such a clause deleted. If unsuccessful in removing the "hold harmless" clause, the pediatrician must check with his or her malpractice carrier to ensure that this clause does not negate the malpractice coverage. Noncoverage by a carrier in this situation must render the clause nonnegotiable because the pediatrician would be shouldering an unacceptable risk.

Another nonnegotiable clause is one that censors physician-patient communication. Termed "gag clauses," these provisions prohibit physicians from fully discussing treatment options with their patients and thereby compromise a physician's ethical and legal duty to the patient. Pediatricians must not sign contracts that contain such provisions.

## EMPLOYEE RETIREMENT INCOME SECURITY ACT OF 1974 (ERISA)

Presently, ERISA laws, which protect self-funded employee benefit plans, prevent many patients from successfully suing their health care entity for negligence. In *Corcoran v United Healthcare*,[4] the court stated that the health care plan did make medical decisions but only "in the context of making a determination about the availability of benefits under the ERISA plan." Under certain conditions ERISA may limit not only the ability of a patient to claim malpractice but also the monetary amounts available from a lawsuit. Recently, however, the ERISA preemption provisions have come under attack and their scope may become limited.

## RESPONSIBILITY OF PEDIATRICIAN IN MANAGED CARE

As managed care continues to expand, so will the legal pitfalls that an individual pediatrician may encounter. It is the responsibility of each pediatrician to keep up with this ever-evolving area of medical care and thereby continue to offer the best medical care possible at the least possible risk to both patients and providers.

COMMITTEE ON MEDICAL LIABILITY, 1995 TO 1996
Mark S. Reuben, MD, Chair
Jan Ellen Berger, MD, MJ
Jeffery I. Berman, MD
Charles H. Deitschel, MD
Ian R. Holzman, MD
Julius Landwirth, MD
Steven M. Selbst, MD

CONSULTANTS
Kenneth V. Heland, JD
    American College of Obstetricians and
    Gynecologists
Holly Myers, JD
    Insurance Consultant

Alain J. Montegut, MD
    American Academy of Family Physicians
Raymond C. Seligson, MD, JD
    Resident Consultant

## REFERENCES

1. Emmons DW, Simon C. *Recent Trends in Managed Care: Socioeconomic Characteristics of Medical Practice.* Chicago, IL: American Medical Association; 1994
2. *Wickline v State of California,* 192 Cal App 3d 1630 (Cal Ct App 1987), *review dismissed, remanded,* 741 P2d 613 (Cal 1987)
3. *Wilson v Blue Cross of Southern California,* 222 Cal App 3d 660 (Cal Ct App 1990)
4. *Corcoran v United Healthcare, Inc,* 965 F 2d 1321 (5th Cir 1992), *cert denied,* 113 S Ct 812 (1992)

# AMERICAN ACADEMY OF PEDIATRICS
## Medicaid Policy Statement (RE9333)

### Committee on Child Health Financing

The American Academy of Pediatrics recognizes the achievements of the Medicaid program in improving access to health care services for poor children. Despite recent legislative expansions to extend eligibility to more poor and disabled children and to broaden the scope of preventive and treatment services in all states, several additional program improvements are needed to eliminate the following barriers to access:

1. Federal and state fiscal crises are creating major roadblocks to Medicaid program implementation and expansion.
2. Thousands of poor children will not be eligible for Medicaid until October 1, 2001.[1]
3. Only a portion of those who are potentially eligible for Medicaid apply for coverage, and many eligible children do not utilize services.
4. Fewer Medicaid funds are available for primary and preventive care because of the increasing need for long-term care services.
5. Early and periodic screening, diagnosis and treatment (EPSDT)/preventive health services are being received by too few children and the implementation of expanded service coverage under EPSDT, granted in 1989, is subject to a great deal of inconsistent state interpretation.
6. Inadequate provider reimbursement reduces children's access to health care services.

The Academy has developed the "Children First" proposal which calls for the elimination of Medicaid and replaces it with a one-class, private insurance system of universal access to health care for all children through age 21 and for all pregnant women.[2] However, until the "Children First" proposal, or a similar health care reform initiative is implemented, the Academy recommends the following policy actions to improve the current Medicaid program.

### I. Eligibility

A. At a minimum all children through age 21 whose family incomes are at or below 185% of the federal poverty level (FPL) should immediately be eligible for Medicaid.
B. All children should be continuously enrolled for a minimum of 1 year regardless of changes in family structure, income, and resources or because of administrative sanctions, and should remain eligible for continuous enrollment for an additional 6 months after an increase in family income if it is less than 300% of the FPL.
C. Presumptive eligibility, currently available only to pregnant women, should be extended to all children so that immediate and temporary Medicaid coverage can be provided until a formal eligibility determination can be made.
D. States should be encouraged to extend coverage to uninsured children by using more generous income and resource methodologies to determine Medicaid eligibility for children allowed under section 1902 (r)(2) of the Medicaid statute.[3]
E. A "buy-in" program in which individuals can purchase health insurance premiums on an income-adjusted basis through Medicaid should be established for children living in families whose income is between current eligibility standards and 300% of the FPL.

### II. Benefits

A. EPSDT-expanded benefit policies in combination with other mandatory and optional benefits should be consistent with the American Academy of Pediatrics' "Scope of Health Care Benefits for Infants, Children and Adolescents Through Age 21 Years"[4] in amount, duration, and scope. Federal and state efforts to assure consistency in the implementation of expanded coverage of diagnostic and treatment services under EPSDT should be strengthened,[5] particularly among managed care providers.
B. EPSDT services should be delivered by a continuing care provider, preferably a pediatrician, according to the American Academy of Pediatrics' "Recommendations for Preventive Pediatric Health Care."[6] If partial screens are performed, arrangements should be made for the patient to receive continuing care.

### III. Financing

A. Entitlement funding should be continued.
B. Financing safeguards should be implemented to assure that funding levels are sufficient to meet children's health care needs under Medicaid. Serious consideration should be given to an alternative financing arrangement to avoid the financial pitfalls associated with Medicaid which relies so heavily on federal and state funding. This could include (1) creating a children's trust similar to the federal trust funds currently used to finance Medicare and Social Security, and (2) dedicating tax revenues as is done with the Presidential Election Campaign fund.
C. States should be given maximum flexibility to raise funds for their portion of the federal-state match.

### IV. Administration

A. States should designate all hospitals, federally qualified health centers, public health clinics, Title V services, Head Start programs, WIC clinics, and, if feasible, other appropriate health care delivery sites as mandatory "outstationing" sites for processing Medicaid applications.
B. Enrollment in managed care arrangements should be carefully designed to assure access to physicians and other health care providers with expertise in delivering preventive, primary, and specialty services for infants, children, and adolescents.

C. Monitoring requirements should be strengthened to evaluate enrollment experience in managed care arrangements as well as access to appropriate pediatric specialists and treatment modalities.

D. Freedom of choice and other regulation waivers should be approved based on their potential to promote increased access and quality of care, and not be determined solely on the basis of their cost containment potential. In addition, in states where enrollment in managed care plans is mandatory, Medicaid beneficiaries should have the freedom to choose among two or more managed health care plans or between managed care plans and participating private and public providers. In areas where only one managed care plan is available, particularly rural areas, families should be able to choose their individual physicians.

E. Reporting burdens and claim form complexity should be minimized through the development of federal claims payment performance standards that promote prompt provider payment, uniform claims billing, and electronic on-line eligibility verification, as well as minimize retroactive claims denials.

F. Uniformly collected claims data, including age, diagnosis, eligibility category, and recipient identification number, should be encouraged.

G. Simplified enrollment procedures and forms, including the development of culturally appropriate materials, should be implemented to increase beneficiary participation.

H. The number of services requiring prior state approval should be minimized.

I. Enforceable federal sanctions should be imposed on those states found to be out of compliance with Medicaid guidelines set by the Omnibus Reconciliation Acts (OBRA) of 1989 and 1990.

J. Each state should develop a Children's Medicaid Action Plan that will define goals to be achieved and establish outcome objectives for access and health status. These plans should be developed in consultation with pediatricians and other primary health care providers, maternal and child health experts, and Medicaid beneficiaries.

## V. Provider Reimbursement

A. All forms of Medicaid reimbursement (eg, capitation, fee-for-service) should be structured to ensure that pediatric services and procedures are available to Medicaid beneficiaries at least to the extent that such services are available to the general population in the same geographic area.

B. Medicaid physician fees for pediatric care should be at least 90% of the usual, customary, or reasonable (UCR) rates or equivalent to those in Medicare, whichever is higher.

C. To alleviate the states' inappropriate use of the Medicare resource-based relative value scale (RBRVS) to pay for pediatric care, an RBRVS for children's services should be approved by the Health Care Financing Administration (HCFA) that takes into account the physical, developmental, and behavioral differences unique to children. It should be similar in scope and detail to the resource-based relative value scale developed for Medicare.

## VI. Cost Containment and Quality Improvement

A. Cost containment is essential, but should not impede access or compromise the quality of care.

B. Quality assurance standards for children's services covered by Medicaid should be developed and monitored by pediatricians. In addition, qualification standards for nonphysicians who are Medicaid providers should be developed.

C. Preventive care for children through health supervision delivered by a continuing care provider, preferably a pediatrician, is the best approach to containing costs.

D. Utilization management programs should not impede access to health care and must include input from pediatricians.

E. The program should encourage delivery of services in the setting that provides quality care at the lowest cost, eg, treatment in the office as opposed to the emergency department.

F. State financial incentives should be structured to minimize fraud and abuse by providers and beneficiaries, and to recover funds from other liable third parties.

COMMITTEE ON CHILD HEALTH FINANCING, 1992 to 1993
Anthony T. Hirsch, MD, Chairman
Stephen Berman, MD
Joseph C. Bogdan, MD
Gilbert A. Buchanan, MD
Robert D. Gross, MD
Norman Lewak, MD
Richard P. Nelson, MD
Edward A. Penn, MD

SECTION LIAISON
Walter B. Greene, MD

## REFERENCES

1. Fox HB, Wicks LB. *1990 Legislative Provisions Affecting Access to Care by Children and Pregnant Women.* Washington, DC: Fox Health Policy Consultants, Inc; 1993
2. American Academy of Pediatrics, *Children First...A Legislative Proposal.* Elk Grove Village, IL: American Academy of Pediatrics; 1991
3. Fox HB. *The Section 1902 (R) (2) Option to Provide Medicaid Eligibility to Additional Children and Pregnant Women.* Washington, DC: Fox Health Policy Consultants; July 1992
4. American Academy of Pediatrics, Committee on Child Health Financing. Scope of health care benefits for infants, children and adolescents through age 21 years. *Pediatrics.* 1993;91:508
5. Fox HB, Wicks LB. *State Implementation of the OBRA '89 EPSDT Amendments.* Washington, DC: Fox Health Policy Consultants; April 8, 1991
6. American Academy of Pediatrics, Committee on Practice and Ambulatory Medicine. Recommendations for preventive pediatric health care. *AAP News.* July 1991;7

# AMERICAN ACADEMY OF PEDIATRICS

## Principles of Child Health Care Financing    (RE9303)

Committee on Child Health Financing

Inequitable financing mechanisms contribute to the current level of preventable mortality and morbidity today among American infants, children, and adolescents. Current financing systems must be improved to maximize access to and ensure the quality of comprehensive pediatric care.

The American Academy of Pediatrics (AAP) advocates universal and insured financial access to quality health care for all pregnant women and infants, children, and adolescents through age 21 years, hereinafter referred to as pregnant women and children. Such insurance should be a comprehensive benefit package which contains preventive care, including immunizations, and acute and chronic care services.

As the public and private sectors and the AAP continue to explore the structure of health care financing, the following principles will be used to evaluate proposed changes.

1. Children's Right to Access to the Health Care System.

   - All pregnant women and children have a right to comprehensive health care.

   - Financial barriers should not prevent pregnant women and children from receiving comprehensive health care.

   - When families are not covered by insurance provided by an employer, purchase of a private plan, or personal means, pregnant women and children should be insured by public funding.

   - Health care financing mechanisms should permit the patient and his/her family to choose a health care professional who provides quality pediatric care, particularly pediatricians whose offices will serve as the medical home and from which referrals would be made only as appropriate.

   - Managed care plans should not restrict access to qualified pediatric primary care or appropriate referral to pediatric subspecialty and inpatient care. All plans should be required to include representatives of all pediatric subspecialties and inpatient facilities having designated pediatric units in their panel of providers.

2. Standards for Equity, Comprehensiveness, and Quality Assurance.

   - Health care financing mechanisms should cover all health care needs of infants, children, and adolescents through age 21 years as defined by the AAP's Scope of Health Care Benefits for Infants, Children and Adolescents Through Age 21 Years.[1]

   - Health care financing mechanisms should include incentives to promote continuity and coordination of care by primary care pediatricians.

   - Health care financing mechanisms should recognize the value of evaluation and management services, care coordination, and performance of medical/surgical procedures.

   - Appropriate mechanisms for quality improvement including assessments of structure, process and outcome, access, and patient satisfaction must be incorporated into all child health financing systems. Such mechanisms must include appropriate peer review.

   - Health insurers should be prohibited from denying coverage through the use of preexisting conditions exclusion clauses or other inappropriate medical underwriting practices.

   - The specifications and limitations of all health financing plans must be stated clearly and be readily understood by all parties.

   - Health care financing mechanisms should be flexible and pluralistic. Fair competition among health financing and delivery plans is desirable. Competing plans should assure access to quality care. There should be standardization of benefits among programs and requirements for administrative efficiencies such as uniform claims forms and payment mechanisms.

   - Regulations governing health care financing should encourage access to quality care.

3. Standards for Cost Containment.

   - Cost containment is essential, but must not impair the quality of care. Physicians must play an important role in ensuring quality in any cost containment process.

   - Responsibility for controlling costs should be shared by patients, providers, payors, and administrators of health care plans.

PEDIATRICS (ISSN 0031 4005). Copyright © 1993 by the American Academy of Pediatrics.

- Financial incentives should be used to encourage systems that promote quality and efficiency.
- Health care financing mechanisms should encourage delivery of services in the most appropriate and least expensive setting (eg, physician office versus emergency department).
- Cost-sharing should not be applied to preventive and/or health supervision services, including immunizations.

COMMITTEE ON CHILD HEALTH FINANCING, 1991 TO 1992
Anthony T. Hirsch, MD, Chairman

Jerold M. Aronson, MD
Stephen Berman, MD
Gilbert A. Buchanan, MD
Katherine S. Lobach, MD
Hays Mitchell, MD
Donald Muirhead, Jr., MD, MPH
Edward A. Penn, MD

## REFERENCE

1. Committee on Child Health Financing, American Academy of Pediatrics. Scope of health care benefits for infants, children, and adolescents through age 21 years. *Pediatrics*. 1993;91:509

# AMERICAN ACADEMY OF PEDIATRICS

## Why Supplemental Security Income Is Important for Children and Adolescents

Committee on Children With Disabilities     (RE9516)

The Supplemental Security Income (SSI) program for children is an important part of the federal government's social benefits program for children with special needs. The SSI program is a nationwide program administered by the Social Security Administration (SSA) that does the following:

- provides monthly cash payments based on family income,
- qualifies the child for Medicaid health care services in many states, and
- assures referral of SSI child beneficiaries into the state Title V Children With Special Health Care Needs program's system of care.

The SSA considers a child to be disabled if:

- the impairment–physical or mental, or chronic medical condition–is as severe as a condition that would keep an adult from working,
- the condition is expected to last a long time or is life threatening, and
- the child is unable to engage in the everyday activities that most children the same age can do.

Congress implemented the children's component of the SSI program in 1974 in recognition that disabled children who live in low-income households are among the most disadvantaged of all Americans and therefore deserve special assistance. The cost of caring for a child with special needs is an especially heavy burden for families with limited resources. The intent of the SSI program is to reduce the additional deleterious environmental effects that a low family income can have on the growth and development of the disabled child and thereby help these children become self-supporting members of society.

The SSI program provides cash benefits. Therefore, parents can decide how best to use these flexible funds to meet the needs of their child, such as for respite care, special equipment, or transportation to the physician's office. These benefits can also offset the potential income of a second working parent, thus allowing a mother or father to provide care for the child at home.

In addition, SSI eligibility automatically qualifies the child for Medicaid in many states. Because the income eligibility requirements for SSI are in general more liberal than those for Medicaid, the SSI program can provide disabled children access to the health care services that they might not otherwise be able to afford. In addition, all state Title V Children With Special Health Care Needs programs assist SSI child beneficiaries to access health and other needed supportive services that may be available through public and private programs.

The SSI rules for determining financial eligibility and disability are very complex. In addition, significant changes have been made recently to the eligibility criteria. The SSI program has never been well understood by many parents, health care providers, and program administrators at the federal, state, and local levels. Although approximately 910 780 children (0 to 21 years of age) were receiving SSI benefits as of June 1994, many more children would receive SSI benefits-if they applied. This statement provides basic information about the SSI program and describes the roles that pediatricians can play in the SSI outreach, application, and disability determination processes.

### FINANCIAL/RESOURCE ELIGIBILITY CRITERIA

The financial and resource eligibility criteria for SSI are extremely complicated. Although there are general guidelines, there are many exceptions. Therefore, the information provided here should be used as a general guide. The income limits for the SSI program are more liberal than some other federal assistance programs, such as Medicaid. For example, in 1994 a family with two parents in the home and two children in addition to the disabled child can earn up to $2800 per month and still be financially eligible for SSI; a family with one parent in the home and two children in addition to the disabled child can earn up to $2354. There are also limits on the amount of total assets (resources), such as jewelry, a savings account, or a checking account, that a family can have. The limit on assets is $2000 if one parent lives in the household and $3000 if two parents live in the household. When the family's assets are calculated, the following are not included: the family home (regardless of its value), household goods and personal effects up to $2000, and, generally, the family car. Additional information about 1994 income limits is included in Appendix A. These income limits are updated periodically.

This statement has been approved by the Council on Child and Adolescent Health.

The recommendations in this policy statement do not indicate an exclusive course of treatment or serve as a standard of medical care. Variations, taking into account individual circumstances, may be appropriate.

PEDIATRICS (ISSN 0031 4005). Copyright © 1995 by the American Academy of Pediatrics.

## THE ZEBLEY DECISION

A significant change in the SSI program resulted from the February 1990 U.S. Supreme Court decision in the case of *Sullivan, Secretary of HHS, v Zebley.* In this decision, the Supreme Court ruled that the procedures used by the SSA to determine the eligibility of children for SSI were unconstitutional.

Before the Zebley decision, there was no assessment of a child applicant's "functional status" as part of the disability determination process. It was this omission that the Supreme Court cited as unconstitutional, because it discriminated against children by requiring them to meet stricter standards than adults to qualify for SSI. Thus, the child's functional status, in addition to diagnosis, became a critical factor in determining eligibility for SSI.

As a result of this ruling, the SSA has done the following:

- contacted and reevaluated children who had been denied benefits between January 1, 1980, and February 11, 1991, based on medical evidence alone (termed the "Zebley class"),
- developed new methods for gathering information about the medical condition and functional status of children,
- worked to improve the ways in which parents receive information about the program and apply for benefits, and
- developed methods for assessing the functional status of children.

The SSA methods for assessing functional status are now more applicable to children and take into consideration the child's ability to perform expected, age-appropriate activities; the impact of multiple conditions; and the child's need for support and assistance from others.

## DETERMINATION OF ELIGIBILITY FOR SSI

### Presumptive Eligibility

If a child has 1 of 13 specific impairments, he or she may be found "presumptively eligible" for disability payments by the SSA field office staff. These 13 conditions are as follows:

- amputation of two limbs;
- amputation of a leg at the hip;
- total blindness;
- total deafness;
- bed confinement or immobility because of a long-standing condition;
- stroke/cerebral vascular accident that occurred more than 3 months ago, with the child having continued marked difficulty in walking or using a hand or arm;
- cerebral palsy, muscular dystrophy or muscular atrophy, and marked difficulty in walking, speaking, or coordinating the hands;
- diabetes with amputation of a foot;
- Down syndrome;
- for a child 7 years and older, severe mental deficiency;
- renal disease requiring dialysis on a regular basis;
- human immunodeficiency virus infection; and
- birth weight less than 1200 g and less than 1 year of age.

A child can be presumptively eligible and receive SSI benefits for up to 6 months while the formal evaluation of eligibility is conducted. The decision of whether the child is presumptively eligible is based in part on the family's statements and on observations of the child by SSA staff members. The SSA staff cannot evaluate medical evidence. The pediatrician who treats a child with 1 of these 13 conditions should provide the parents with a statement about the diagnosis and the severity of the child's disabling condition. Parents need to know that they can request presumptive eligibility for their child based on this statement.

### Disability Determination

The SSA does not make disability determinations directly. Rather, it has a contract with a state Disability Determination Services (DDS) agency to perform this function. State DDS agencies operate under federal regulations and instructions issued by the SSA. Once the SSA determines that the child is a U.S. citizen and appears to qualify financially, information about the child's disability and a list of additional sources of information are sent to the DDS unit. (Additional information about citizen/residency requirements is included in Appendix B.) The DDS agency uses a team comprised of a disability examiner and a medical or psychological professional to decide whether the child is eligible, based on the available written information.

The disability examiner must develop a complete medical and functional history for the child for at least the 12 months preceding the application for SSI. Staff of the DDS do not examine the child or meet with the child or family. Because the determination made by the state DDS unit is based on written information, it is important that pediatricians provide complete, detailed data in response to requests for information from the DDS.

Therefore, the pediatrician's medical report in support of a child's application for SSI should do the following:

- Refer to the SSA's childhood "Listing of Impairments" and use the specific terms and reference the specific clinical tests included in the listings. The listing contains criteria for evaluating the impairments of children (younger than 18 years), ie, mental and physical symptoms, signs, and/or laboratory findings, and includes 66 childhood diseases and disorders. These listings, however, have been criticized for omitting many disabling conditions. (A copy of the "Disability Evaluation Under Social Security" may be obtained from the SSA Office of Public Affairs, Public Information Distribution Center, P.O. Box 17743, Baltimore, MD 21235; telephone 410–965–0945, fax 410-965-0696).
- Include a medical history of the child (for at least

the previous 12 months).

- Provide complete, detailed clinical findings (eg, the results of physical, intelligence, developmental, and mental status examinations).
- Include complete, detailed laboratory findings (eg, blood pressure, radiographic films).
- Specify the diagnosis (statement of disease/injury based on signs and symptoms).
- Review treatment(s) prescribed with response and prognosis.
- State the probable duration of the impairment.
- Include an assessment of the child's physical or mental abilities to function independently, appropriately, and effectively in an age-appropriate manner and to perform age-appropriate daily activities.
- Describe the nature and limiting effects of the impairment(s) on the child's ability to function independently, appropriately, and effectively in an age-appropriate manner and to perform age-appropriate daily activities.

If the available information provided by those who treat the child is insufficient for determining disability, the DDS can arrange for a consultative examination at the SSA's expense by the child's treating physician, or, if the treating physician is unable or unwilling to conduct the examination, by an independent physician. On the basis of all the available information, the DDS follows a four-step process ("sequential evaluation") to make a determination. The steps of this process and the decision criteria are described in the Figure and given in detail below. The DDS then informs the SSA of the decision, which

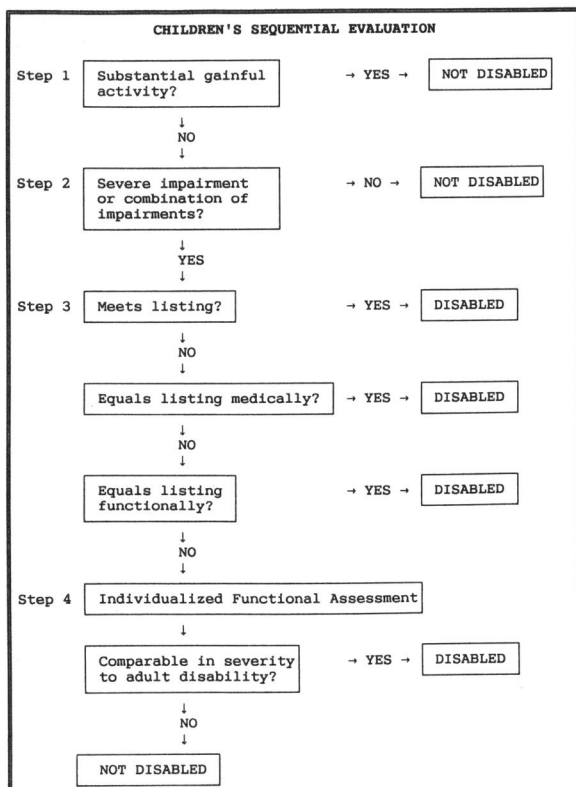

Figure. Children's Sequential Evaluation.

is given to the parents in writing. The process of determining disability can take 2 to 3 months. If the application is rejected, the parents have the right to appeal the decision.

### THE FOUR-STEP EVALUATION PROCESS

In step 1, the examiner determines whether the child is engaged in Substantial Gainful Activity, ie, work. If the applicant engages in Substantial Gainful Activity, the claim is rejected. If the child does not engage in such activity, step 2 is begun.

In step 2, the examiner determines, based on the available documentation, whether the applicant has a severe impairment or combination of impairments. Severe is defined as more than a minimal or slight limitation in a child's ability to function independently, appropriately, and effectively in an age-appropriate manner. If the examiner determines that the impairment is severe, or if there is doubt about the severity or the effect of the impairment on the child's functioning, step 3 begins. If the applicant has a minimal or slight limitation impairment, the claim is rejected.

In step 3, the examiner determines whether the child's impairment is the same as ("meets") or is either medically or functionally equivalent in severity to ("equals") one of the conditions on the SSA's "Listing of Impairments."

An examiner will find that a child meets a listing only when the symptoms, signs, and laboratory findings meet the findings included in the criteria for that listed impairment. If an examiner finds that a child meets a listing, then the child is determined to be disabled and is eligible for SSI benefits. If the child does not meet a listing, the examiner must determine whether the child's impairment is medically equivalent in severity to any listed impairment. If it is not, the examiner must determine whether the impairment is functionally equivalent in severity to a listed impairment.

An examiner must determine whether the available documentation indicates that a child's impairment or combination of impairments exhibits signs, symptoms, and laboratory findings that are of equal medical significance or severity to the listed criteria. If the child's impairment is judged to be medically equivalent to a listed impairment, he or she is classified as disabled. If the child's impairment is not judged to be medically equivalent, the examiner must determine whether the impairment is functionally equivalent in severity to a listed impairment. For example, according to listing 106.02D, a child who has had a kidney transplantation should be considered disabled for at least 1 year after the transplantation. Although not specifically listed, a child with disability from a heart transplantation should be found "equivalent to a kidney transplant because it has a similar impact on a child's ability to function in an age-appropriate manner" (Clark and Manes, 1992, chapter 12, page 6). The SSA rules and regulations (20 C.F.R. § 416.926a[d]) provide 15 examples of impairments that are functionally equivalent to those in the listings. If the child's impairment is judged to be functionally equivalent to a listed impairment, he or she is classified as disabled. If it is not, then the examiner must complete an Individualized Functional Assessment.

Step 4, the process of Individualized Functional Assessment, is the major modification to the SSI regulations by the SSA in response to the Zebley decision. The examiner must determine whether the impairments limit the child's ability, as much as they would an adult's ability, to function independently, appropriately, and effectively in an age-appropriate manner. The SSA's definition of "comparable severity" was expanded to take into consideration that if the manifestations of impairments in children are age related, then the evidence needed to evaluate disability appropriately is age related. The new SSI regulations specify the following age groups:

- newborns and young infants (birth to age 1 year),
- older infants and toddlers (ages 1 to 3 years),
- preschool children (ages 3 to 6 years),
- school-age children (ages 6 to 12 years),
- young adolescents (ages 12 to 16 years), and
- older adolescents (ages 16 to 18 years).

When evaluating the functional status of children aged 0 to 16 years, DDS examiners focus on the following:

- cognition (the child's ability to learn),
- communication skills (the child's ability to receive, understand, and express messages; with respect to speech, audibility, intelligibility, and efficiency of speech production),
- motor skills (the child's ability to use his or her body, hands, and feet in gross and fine motions),
- social skills (the child's ability to form, develop, and sustain relationships with other people on a personal and social basis), and
- personal/behavioral patterns, which refer to activities and behaviors entailed in the following: self-help, such as feeding and dressing; self-regulation, such as maintaining proper nutrition and sleep; self-improvement, such as increasing self-help behavior through learning new skills; self-protection, such as taking necessary safety precautions; and self-control, such as adapting to changes in the environment or an activity, or controlling impulsive or aggressive behaviors that could result in self-harm.

For evaluation of the functional status of infants, information should be provided about the child's physical and emotional responses to stimuli. For children older than 3 years, concentration, persistence, and pace in the completion of tasks should be evaluated. For older adolescents aged 16 and 17 years, school and work-like activities and the ability to function in a work setting are relevant factors.

As part of the Individualized Functional Assessment, the disability examiner must develop a complete medical and functional history for the child for at least the 12 months preceding the application for SSI. In determining the child's functional capacity, the examiner must also consider the impact of the following.

*Chronic Illness.* Detailed descriptive information should be provided if hospitalizations are so extended or frequent that they interfere with overall functioning, or if the frequency and/or effects of outpatient care significantly interfere with the child's daily activities.

*Medication.* Detailed descriptive information should be provided if medications and/or side effects cause or contribute to a child's functional limitations.

*Supportive and Structured Settings.* Detailed descriptive information should be provided as to how a child's symptoms are controlled or reduced by a highly structured or supportive environment, and whether the child can function independently, appropriately, and effectively in an age-appropriate manner outside of this environment.

*Assistive Devices, Appliances, and Technology and Special Support Services.* Detailed descriptive information should be provided if special devices or services provide some improvement without restoring adequate functioning, or if they themselves impose limitations.

*Frequent and Ongoing Therapeutic Intervention.* Detailed descriptive information should be provided if the multidisciplinary therapies that the child receives interrupt school or home activities and interfere with the child's development and age-appropriate functioning.

Although the information provided to the DDS by pediatricians is critical to the efficient, accurate determination of disability, pediatricians and other professionals generally do not describe a child's physical status and impairments using the criteria listed above. A physician's declaration that a child is disabled is not sufficient evidence for the DDS to determine a child eligible for SSI benefits. The SSA regulations require that the DDS perform a functional assessment of physically impaired children that relies on the pediatrician's providing information according to the factors listed above. Reports should use the specific terms and reference the specific clinical tests included in the "Listings of Impairments." In addition, when possible, formal test results regarding the child's functioning and development should be provided in terms of percentiles, percentages, standard deviations, or the fraction or percentage of the child's chronological age.

### WHAT TO TELL FAMILIES ABOUT SSI APPLICATION, DISABILITY DETERMINATION, AND APPEALS PROCEDURES

Appendix C gives detailed information about how families can apply for SSI benefits for a disabled child.

### CONCLUSION AND RECOMMENDATIONS

Pediatricians, individually and through state chapters of the American Academy of Pediatrics, can play a critical role in helping to ensure that all eligible children receive the SSI cash and associated benefits to which they are entitled. These efforts should include:

- providing information about the SSI program to families;
- increasing their knowledge about the SSI program and providing specific, detailed reports to the DDS in support of children's applications for SSI benefits; and
- advocating for better reimbursement and improved methods for providing reports to the DDS.
- The SSA has a variety of brochures designed to inform families about the SSI program. Physicians and state chapters should contact their local SSA field office to develop ways for making this information available through physicians' offices.

The SSA and state DDS units have designated the staff responsible for educating the professional community about the SSI program. The chapters of the American Academy of Pediatrics should invite the staffs of the SSA and DDS to participate in local and state-wide educational meetings and workshops. This will help ensure that the pediatric community is informed about the SSI program and skilled in providing medical evidence to support their patients' applications for SSI benefits. Such efforts can also help to develop working relationships between these agencies and the pediatric community.

Reimbursement for reports provided by physicians to the DDS is generally considered inadequate. State chapters can advocate for change in the reimbursement schedule and can also work with the state DDS unit to develop more efficient methods for providing reports. Some state DDS units have implemented a system whereby local physicians can call the DDS office and dictate their report on a child applicant. The DDS takes responsibility for transcribing this information and entering it into the child's application. Some state DDS agencies also provide report outlines to help focus the information on the pediatrician's report. Other agencies also use a professional advisory board. State chapters can advocate for the use or expansion of such a board to ensure that there is a good working relationship between the agency and the pediatric community.

These activities will help ensure that the SSI program is implemented more fully and that low-income, disabled children and their families receive the support and benefits they need.

## APPENDIX A: SSI SCREENING—PARENT TO CHILD DEEMING

**TABLE.** Monthly Deeming Breakeven Points for Federal SSI Payment, Effective January 1, 1994, Through December 31, 1994*

| | (All income must be below the following amounts) | | | |
| No. of Ineligible CHILDREN | All Income Is Work Income | | All Income Is Nonwork Income† | |
| | 1 Parent | 2 Parents‡ | 1 Parent | 2 Parents‡ |
|---|---|---|---|---|
| 0 | $1908 | $2354 | $ 931 | $1154 |
| 1 | $2131 | $2577 | $1154 | $1377 |
| 2 | $2354 | $2800 | $1377 | $1600 |
| 3 | $2577 | $3023 | $1600 | $1823 |
| 4 | $2800 | $3246 | $1823 | $2046 |
| 5 | $3023 | $3469 | $2046 | $2269 |
| 6 | $3246 | $3692 | $2269 | $2492 |

* Notes:
  1. These income amounts refer to eligibility for the federal benefit only. Add the applicable state supplementation amount to these amounts.
  2. All amounts assume that all children have no income and there is only one eligible child in the household. In any other case, refer to SSA.
  3. For each additional ineligible child in the household (over six ineligible children), add $218 to the amount shown.
  4. This chart does not work if the ineligible parent(s) has/have both work and nonwork income.
† Common types of income not counted in deeming:
  1. Public income maintenance payments.
  2. Income used to figure public income maintenance payments.
  3. Foster care payments.
  4. Food stamps, Department of Agriculture donated foods.
  5. Income set aside under a plan for self-support.
  6. Income used to pay court-ordered or Title IV-D support payments.
  7. The value of in-kind support and maintenance.
‡ For a two-parent household, even if only one parent has income.

## APPENDIX B: SSI CITIZENSHIP AND RESIDENCY ELIGIBILITY CRITERIA

To be eligible for SSI, a child must be a U.S. citizen or a naturalized citizen. The SSA defines a child as an individual who is younger than 18 years or younger than 22 years and a student, not married, and not the "head of a household." Children authorized to remain in the U.S. by the Immigration and Naturalization Service may also qualify. The child must also reside in one of the 50 states, the District of Columbia, or the northern Mariana Islands. Children living in Puerto Rico, Guam, and the U.S. Virgin Islands may be U.S. citizens but do not meet the SSI requirements for residency. The exception is children of military personnel who are assigned overseas duty.

## APPENDIX C: WHAT TO TELL FAMILIES ABOUT SSI APPLICATION, DISABILITY DETERMINATION, AND APPEALS PROCEDURES

### How to Apply

To apply for SSI benefits for a disabled child, a parent must complete, sign, and file a form that can be obtained by either

- visiting the local SSA field office or
- calling the SSA's toll-free number (1–800–772–1213) to make an appointment for a telephone interview.

### Telephone Interview

If parents make an appointment for a telephone interview by calling the toll-free number, they should be contacted by staff of the SSA's telephone screening service. The interviewer will provide general information to parents about the medical, disability, and functional criteria that are used in determining eligibility for SSI. Information about disability criteria is provided to help parents decide whether they should proceed with the application process. The SSA prefers that parents use the telephone screening process because, according to the SSA, it is more efficient for both the parents and the SSA.

Parents need to know the following:

- the telephone line is often busy, but they should keep trying;
- the SSA interviewer will gather information about family income, financial resources, and the child's citizenship;
- on the basis of the above information, the interviewer will indicate whether it appears (or does not appear) that the child is financially eligible for SSI;
- the interviewer will ask whether they want to file an application for the child;
- they have a right to request and file an application even if it does not appear that the child qualifies financially;
- application forms will be sent by mail to their home;
- the telephone interviewer should not suggest that the child does (or does not) appear to meet the SSI disability criteria;
- the date of the telephone interview serves as the "protected filing date" and, if the child is found to be eligible for SSI, benefits will be paid back to this date;
- they should keep a record of all contacts with the SSA, including the date and the person with whom they spoke;
- the process of determining disability can take 2 to 3 months; and
- financial eligibility for young adults 18 years or

older is based only on what they own and/or earn; family income/assets are not considered.

### Applying at the SSA Field Office

If parents choose to go to a local SSA field office, they should call the local office or the toll-free number to make an appointment. This will ensure that an SSA staff person will be available to take the application and will reduce the amount of time the parents have to wait when filing an application.

If parents have a problem gathering all of the required information, they should still go to the SSA field office to begin the application process to establish a protected filing date. When the SSA has the needed information about family income and financial resources, financial eligibility for SSI will be determined.

COMMITTEE ON CHILDREN WITH DISABILITIES, 1994 TO 1995
James Perrin, MD, Chair
Gerald Erenberg, MD
Robert La Camera, MD
John A. Nackashi, MD
John R. Poncher, MD
Virginia Randall, MD
Renee C. Wachtel, MD
W. Daniel Williamson, MD
Philip R. Ziring, MD

LIAISON REPRESENTATIVES
Debbie Gaebler, MD
Connie Garner, RN, MSN, EdD, United States Department of Education Programs
Joseph G. Hollowell, MD, Centers for Disease Control and Prevention, Center for Environmental Health and Injury Control
Merle McPherson, MD, Maternal and Child Health Bureau, Department of Health and Human Services

SECTION LIAISON
Harry Gewanter, MD, Section on Rheumatology

CONSULTANT
John Reiss, PhD
Institute for Child Health Policy, University of Florida

### Suggested Readings

Clark J, Manes J. *Advocate's Guide to SSI for Children*. Washington, DC: Bazelon Center for Mental Health Law; 1992

Force J, Grason H. Social Security Supplemental Security Income (SSI) program for disabled children. In: *Developmental Handicaps: Prevention and Treatment IV*. Silver Spring, MD: American Association of University Affiliated Programs; 1987

Fox H, Greaney A. *Disabled Children's Access to Supplemental Security Income and Medicaid Benefits*. Washington, DC: Fox Health Policy Consultants; 1988

Perrin J, Stein REK. Reinterpreting disability: changes in supplemental security income for children. *Pediatrics*. 1991;87:1047–1051

Reiss J, Siderits P, eds. *SSI Handbook*. Gainesville, FL: Institute for Child Health Policy; 1991

Reiss J, Talaga E. *SSInsights: A Curriculum on Providing SSI Medical and Other Evidence*. Gainesville, FL: Institute for Child Health Policy; 1995

Social Security Administration. *Disability Evaluation Under Social Security*. Publication no. 64–039. Baltimore, MD: SSA; 1994

Social Security Administration. *A Guide for Treating Physicians and Other Health Care Professionals*. Publication no. 64–084. Baltimore, MD: SSA; 1993

*Sullivan v Zebley*, 88–1377 (U.S. Supreme Court, 20 Feb 1990)

# AMERICAN ACADEMY OF PEDIATRICS

## Ethics and the Care of Critically Ill Infants and Children

Committee on Bioethics        (RE9624)

**ABSTRACT.** The ability to provide life support to ill children who, not long ago, would have died despite medicine's best efforts challenges pediatricians and families to address profound moral questions. Our society has been divided about extending the life of some patients, especially newborns and older infants with severe disabilities. The American Academy of Pediatrics (AAP) supports individualized decision making about life-sustaining medical treatment for all children, regardless of age. These decisions should be jointly made by physicians and parents, unless good reasons require invoking established child protective services to contravene parental authority. At this time, resource allocation (rationing) decisions about which children should receive intensive care resources should be made clear and explicit in public policy, rather than be made at the bedside.

Since the advent of means for supporting newborns with respiratory distress, neonatal and pediatric intensive care has helped tens of thousands of children survive life-threatening illness and the rigors of major surgical intervention. For more than a decade, however, many responsible for the health care of children have debated the appropriateness of applying life-sustaining medical technology (LSMT) to all critically ill children. (The term LSMT here applies to methods of supporting life typically applied in intensive care units, such as the use of ventilators and mechanical or pharmacologic support of circulation. The term critically ill here refers to disorders requiring such LSMT. Both terms defy precise definition.) As a recent AAP policy statement[1] on forgoing LSMT notes, the value of such therapy may be uncertain, especially when first considered. Good medical practice may favor initiation of LSMT until clarification of the clinical situation and relevant ethical values can occur. Much discussion has focused on highly visible "selective nontreatment of handicapped infants"[2] and the responses of the federal government, now known colloquially as the "Baby Doe" rules.[3,4] In the last few years, clinicians and the public also have become increasingly concerned about the high costs, in terms of money, time, and psychosocial consequences, of neonatal and pediatric intensive care.

### NEWBORNS AND INFANTS

Much controversy has surrounded the treatment of newborns and older infants with readily identifiable medical problems, including genetic disorders, malformations and deformations, and, to some extent, extreme prematurity and/or low birth weight. Scientific understanding and improved technology have permitted reductions in mortality for infants affected by an enlarging list of conditions. A better appreciation of what can be done to help many infants with disabilities and social considerations of fairness have led to the application of life-saving medical interventions to critically ill newborns and infants who, not long ago, physicians might not have treated vigorously. Concern that some infants, eg, those with Down syndrome and gastrointestinal obstruction, received insufficient treatment led to the federal legislation (the 1984 Child Abuse Amendments) and regulations that sought to ensure appropriate medical therapy for all disabled infants.

Looking back, the measures to prevent undue discrimination against disabled infants seem to have produced at least two unintended consequences. First, it seems that many persons in the health care and child advocacy professions, along with the general public, misunderstand the various federal and other legal requirements regarding treatment decisions for infants with critical illnesses.[5–7] Thus, misconceptions about the Baby Doe rules may have become de facto benchmarks for treatment decisions about critically ill newborns and older infants. Second, attention concentrated on saving the lives of infants, some with permanent, severe disabilities or neurodegenerative disorders, has hampered sufficient attention to the possible overuse of LSMT.

With regard to the first point, the actual language of the 1984 Child Abuse Amendments may permit more physician discretion than some realize. Although the law mandates provision of LSMT to most seriously ill infants, it does provide for exceptions in the case of permanent unconsciousness, "futile" treatment, and "virtually futile" therapy that imposes excessive burdens on the infant. Physicians, with parental agreement, may even forgo giving hydration and nutrition when they think these measures are not "appropriate." (Quoted words and phrases come directly from the law.[3])

With regard to the second point, possible overuse of LSMT, several book-length studies,[8–11] one personal account from parents,[12] and recent essays by pioneering neonatologists[13,14] have suggested that modern newborn care may, at times, constitute overtreatment. Articles for the general public have communicated the same message.[15–17] As previously noted, after the Child Abuse Amendments of 1984, two reports of a survey of neonatologists[5,6] indicated

PEDIATRICS (ISSN 0031 4005). Copyright © 1996 by the American Academy of Pediatrics.

that many who specialize in the care of sick new-borns believe they are legally constrained to provide LSMT to infants, even when their medical judgments and the views of the parents concur that withholding treatment is preferable.

Although many would like to have simply interpreted and easily applied substantive standards for clinical decisions about critically ill infants, medical and moral complexity make such rules imprudent. Scientific uncertainty regarding outcome continues in the neonatal intensive care unit. Some very tiny infants with documented brain insults, such as those that may occur with periventricular hemorrhage, defy expectations and survive with no apparent clinical deficits. Available evidence, however, continues to indicate that the decreased mortality brought about by neonatal intensive care has been accompanied by increased morbidity, ie, serious mental and physical limitations among survivors that impose burdens on affected children and their families.[18,19] These factors also play legitimate roles in decision making.[20,21]

A few well-publicized cases in the early 1980s led some to conclude that physicians and parents commonly denied beneficial treatment to imperiled newborns. However, no reliable evidence that decisions endangering children have been widespread exists. Most cases of lethal nontreatment seem to have involved infants with trisomy 21 and myelomeningocele.[22-24] However, by the early 1980s professional and public views about infants with Down syndrome and spina bifida had generally shifted to favor treatment.[25] This view is supported by results from a survey of pediatricians done in Massachusetts in the mid-1980s.[24]

The AAP supports parental involvement in decisions about imperiled infants from the earliest possible moment. Obstetricians and pediatricians need to inform and counsel parents about available options when prenatal diagnostic procedures identify disorders in fetuses. Women may legitimately decide about the treatment they and their fetuses receive.[26,27] Once parturition occurs, parents continue to have a vital role in decision making under the presumption that they accept responsibility for nurturing the infant and providing reasonable care.[28]

The AAP believes that parents and physicians should make reasoned decisions together about critically ill infants using the principles of informed parental permission recently articulated by the AAP.[29] Such decisions should consider the benefits and burdens of treatment alternatives. Physicians should remember that many parents want a strong role in these decisions[30] and that parents may bring values to the process that differ sharply from those of the physician. In rare instances, as required by law and sound ethical standards, it may be necessary to invoke established child protective mechanisms if parents wish to forgo LSMT, physicians disagree, and the parties cannot resolve their differences with help from subspecialists, ethics consultants, or ethics committees.

## CHILDREN BEYOND INFANCY

As with infants, two basic questions arise in the care of children beyond the first year: Which values and whose authority ought to govern in medical treatment decisions about the critically ill? Published court cases indicate that parents have been permitted to exercise broad discretion when acting on their children's behalf,[31-36] even when court-appointed guardians ad litem or other counsel opposed the parental choice.[37-39] Laws in some states permit parents to execute advance directives on behalf of minors (Choice and Dying. State laws regarding end-of-life decision making for minors. New York, NY: Choice and Dying; September 1995:1–2).[40] In addition to according due respect to the beliefs, feelings, and needs of the family as expressed by parents, as children get older and acquire cognitive skill, experience, and emotional maturity, their individual views deserve careful consideration. Sensitive clinicians and parents acknowledged this in the professional literature as long as 20 years ago.[41]

In the realm of pediatric critical care, the North American literature provides sparse evidence of systematic approaches to limiting LSMT.[42,43] The pediatric intensive care unit, however, unlike the neonatal intensive care unit, has not been the focus of bureaucratic or political debate and action. Pediatric intensivists and their colleagues and consultants in ethics have tended to make decisions about discontinuing LSMT similar to the way clinicians, loved ones, ethicists, and the courts make such decisions for incompetent adult patients.[44,45]

## RESOURCE ALLOCATION AND DECISIONS TO LIMIT LSMT

Recently, concerns about the high cost of critical care have led to attempts to manage critical care resources through the use of quantitative indicators of prognosis.[46-51] Some physicians, administrators, and planners would like to use increasingly accurate statistical predictors of outcome to exclude patients from receiving intensive care services. Indeed, population-based mathematical tools may prove helpful in evaluating the effectiveness of various interventions, in comparing outcomes of similar treatments used at different sites, and in informing parents of the probability of the outcome of treatment. Such studies, however, have an important inherent limitation—their results apply to groups of patients, not individuals. In the absence of perfect outcome prediction (100% survival or death, based on experience with large numbers of patients), statistical indicators cannot tell clinicians which particular patient will die or live (and with what residual problems). Moreover, even overwhelming odds of success or failure of treatment cannot take into account the complex values that individuals, including patients, family members, physicians, and other health care providers, bring to a treatment decision. Therefore, the AAP opposes the use of these formulas as the principal determinants of whether individual patients receive intensive care.

The controversy over the usefulness of critical care

resources has been most poignantly highlighted by public debates about futile medical treatment.[52–56] In these discussions, physicians and other care givers have demonstrated concern that medical resources are being used inappropriately and that continued treatment violates deeply held beliefs about what properly constitutes professional activities. Others feel that professional objections to so-called futile treatment masks prejudices about those who are disabled, who come from disadvantaged social groups, or who are dying.

The AAP thinks that judgments about which diagnostic categories of patients should receive or be denied intensive care based on considerations of resource use are social policy deliberations and should be made after considerable public discussion, not ad hoc at the bedside.

## CONCLUSIONS

Our society has reached a consensus that some critically ill infants previously denied treatment should receive advanced medical and surgical care. A large majority of physicians and other persons agree that most infants with Down syndrome with gastrointestinal obstruction and most infants with myelomeningocele should have surgery and other treatment they need.

There is less agreement, however, about how much treatment to provide other critically ill infants and children. Medical and public controversy still rages about the appropriate limits, if any, to place on the treatment of extremely low birth weight and premature infants, about infants with hypoplastic left heart syndrome,[57] about children with chromosomal abnormalities with known very limited life spans, about infants with complex congenital abnormalities, and about children in the final stages of terminal cancer or other fatal chronic disorders. Many think that laws, regulations, and government policies have unduly constrained parents and physicians from exercising reasonable judgments about whether to forgo LSMT.

A judicial and legislative consensus has developed that the values of patients, rather than those of physicians or policy makers, should determine the extent of the application of LSMT.[58] As noted, some states have empowered proxy decision makers to execute advance directives regarding LSMT on behalf of minors. Legislation and regulation about disabled infants conflict with the legal trends governing all other patients. In the absence of compelling evidence that infants require special legal protection, the AAP thinks that parents of newborns should have the same decision-making authority they have with older children.

Limited resources may require equitable limits on medical treatment. Such restrictions require careful consideration of their social, cultural, and economic consequences and deserve to be made at a public policy level, not at the bedside.

## RECOMMENDATIONS

1. Decisions about critical care for newborns, infants, and children should be made similarly and with informed parental permission.
2. Physicians should recommend the provision or forgoing of critical care services based on the projected benefits and burdens of treatment, recognizing that parents may perceive and value these benefits and burdens differently from medical professionals.
3. Decisions to forgo critical care services on the grounds of resource limitations, generally speaking, are not clinical decisions, and physicians should avoid such "bedside rationing."

However, because many in the American public think that our health care system spends excessively on critical care services, society should engage in a thoroughgoing debate about the economic, cultural, religious, social, and moral consequences of imposing limits on which patients should receive intensive care.

COMMITTEE ON BIOETHICS, 1995 TO 1996
Joel E. Frader, MD, Chairperson
Lucy S. Crain, MD
Kathryn L. Moseley, MD
Robert M. Nelson, MD
Ian H. Porter, MD
Felipe E. Vizcarrondo, MD

LIAISON REPRESENTATIVES
Watson A. Bowes, MD
    American College of Obstetricians and
    Gynecologists
Alessandra Kazura, MD
    American Academy of Child and Adolescent
    Psychiatry
Ernest Krug, MD
    American Board of Pediatrics

SECTION LIAISON
Donna A. Caniano, MD
    Section on Surgery

LEGAL CONSULTANT
Nancy M. P. King

## REFERENCES

1. American Academy of Pediatrics, Committee on Bioethics. Guidelines on forgoing life-sustaining medical treatment. *Pediatrics.* 1994;93:532–536
2. Weir RF. *Selective Nontreatment of Handicapped Newborns: Moral Dilemmas in Neonatal Medicine.* New York: Oxford University Press; 1992
3. US Child Abuse Protection and Treatment Amendments of 1984. Pub L No. 98-457
4. Child abuse and neglect prevention and treatment program: final rule. 50 *Federal Register* 14878–14901
5. Kopelman LM, Irons TG, Kopelman AE. Neonatologists judge the "Baby Doe" regulations. *N Engl J Med.* 1988;318:677–683
6. Kopelman LM, Kopelman AE, Irons TG. Neonatologists, pediatricians, and the Supreme Court criticize the "Baby Doe" regulations. In: Caplan AL, Blank RH, Merrick JC, eds. *Compelled Compassion: Government Intervention in the Treatment of Critically Ill Newborns.* Totowa, NJ: Humana Press; 1992:237–266
7. Frader J. Review of compelled compassion. *N Engl J Med.* 1992;327:824
8. Guillemin JH, Holmstrom LL. *Mixed Blessings: Intensive Care for Newborns.* New York: Oxford University Press; 1986
9. Frohock FM. *Special Care: Medical Decisions at the Beginning of Life.* Chicago, IL: University of Chicago Press; 1986
10. Bosk CL. *All God's Mistakes: Genetic Counseling in a Pediatric Hospital.* Chicago, IL: University of Chicago Press; 1992
11. Anspach RR. *Deciding Who Lives: Fateful Choices in the Intensive-Care Nursery.* Berkeley, CA: University of California Press; 1993

12. Stinson R, Stinson P. *The Long Dying of Baby Andrew.* Boston, MA: Little, Brown & Co; 1992

13. Silverman A. Overtreatment of neonates? A personal retrospective. *Pediatrics.* 1992;90:971–976

14. Stahlman MT. Ethical issues in the nursery: priorities versus limits. *J Pediatr.* 1990;116:167–170

15. Kolata G. Parents of tiny infants find care choices are not theirs. *New York Times.* September 30, 1991:A1

16. Brody JE. A quality of life determined by a baby's size. *New York Times.* October 1, 1991:A1

17. Quindlen A. Crimes against the smallest of children. *New York Times.* January 29, 1992:A21

18. Paneth N, Stark RI. Cerebral palsy and mental retardation in relation to indicators of perinatal asphyxia. *Am J Obstet Gynecol.* 1983;147:960–966

19. Blank RH. Rationing medicine in the neonatal intensive care unit (NICU). In: Caplan AL, Blank RH, Merrick JC, eds. *Compelled Compassion: Government Intervention in the Treatment of Critically Ill Newborns.* Totowa, NJ: Humana Press; 1992:97–103

20. Strong C. The neonatologist's duty to patient and parents. *Hastings Cent Rep.* 1984;14:10–16

21. Hardwig J. What about the family? *Hastings Cent Rep.* 1990;20:5–10

22. Lantos J. Baby Doe five years later: implications for child health. *N Engl J Med.* 1987;317:444–447

23. Todres ID, Krane D, Howell MC, Shannon DC. Pediatricians' attitudes affecting decision making in defective newborns. *Pediatrics.* 1977;60:197–201

24. Todres ID, Guilleman J, Grodin MA, Batten D. Life-saving therapy for newborns: a questionnaire survey in the state of Massachusetts. *Pediatrics.* 1988;81:643–649

25. Caplan AL. Hard cases make bad law: the legacy of the Baby Doe controversy. In: Caplan AL, Blank RH, Merrick JC, eds. *Compelled Compassion: Government Intervention in the Treatment of Critically Ill Newborns.* Totowa, NJ: Humana Press; 1992:105–122

26. Board of Trustees, American Medical Association. Legal interventions during pregnancy. *JAMA.* 1990;264:2663–2670

27. Committee on Ethics, American College of Obstetricians and Gynecologists. *Patient Choice: Maternal-Fetal Conflict.* Washington, DC: American College of Obstetricians and Gynecologists; 1987. ACOG Committee opinion 55

28. *Bowen v American Hospital Association,* 106 S Ct 2101 (1986)

29. Committee on Bioethics, American Academy of Pediatrics. Informed consent, parental permission, and assent in pediatric practice. *Pediatrics.* 1995;95:314–317

30. Harrison H. The principles for family-centered neonatal care. *Pediatrics.* 1993;92:643–650

31. *In re PVW,* 424 S2d 1015 (La 1982)

32. *In re Crum,* 580 NE2d 876 (Ohio Probate Ct 1991)

33. *In re Lawrance,* 579 NE 2d633 (Ind 1991)

34. *Newmark v Williams,* 588 A2d 1108 (Del 1991)

35. *In re Rosebush,* 491 NW2d 633 (Mich App 1992)

36. *In re "Baby K,"* 16 F3d 590 (4th Cir 1994)

37. *In re CA,* 603 NE2d 1171 (Ill App 1992)

38. *Guardianship of Doe,* 583 NE2d 1263 (Mass 1992)

39. *Care and Protection of Beth,* 587 NE2d 1377 (Mass 1992)

40. Jefferson LS, White BC, Louis PT, Brody BA, King DD, Roberts CE. Use of the Natural Death Act in pediatric patients. *Crit Care Med.* 1991;19:901–905

41. Schowalter J, Ferholt J, Mann N. The adolescent patient's decision to die. *Pediatrics.* 1973;51:97–103

42. Lantos JD, Berger AC, Zucker AR. Do-not-resuscitate orders in a children's hospital. *Crit Care Med.* 1993;21:52–55

43. Leikin S. A proposal concerning decisions to forgo life-sustaining treatment for young people. *J Pediatr.* 1989;115:17–22

44. Frader J. Ethics in pediatric intensive care. In: Fuhrman BP, Zimmerman JJ, eds. *Pediatric Critical Care.* St Louis, MO: Mosby-Year Book, Inc; 1992:7–15

45. Glover JJ, Holbrook PR. Ethical considerations. In: Holbrook PR, ed. *Textbook of Pediatric Critical Care.* Philadelphia, PA: WB Saunders Co; 1993:1124–1130

46. Knaus WA, Wagner DP, Lynn J. Short-term mortality predictions for critically ill hospitalized adults: science and ethics. *Science.* 1991;254:389–394

47. Knaus WA, Wagner DP, Draper EA, et al. The APACHE III prognostic system: risk prediction of hospital mortality for critically ill hospitalized adults. *Chest.* 1991;100:1619–1636

48. Pollack MM, Ruttiman UE, Getson PR. Pediatric risk of mortality (PRISM) score. *Crit Care Med.* 1988;16:1110–1116

49. Pollack MM, Getson PR. Pediatric critical care cost containment: combined actuarial and clinical program. *Crit Care Med.* 1991;19:12–20

50. Tyson J, Wright E, Malloy M, Wright L. How predictable is the outcome and care of ventilated extreme low birth weight (ELBW <1000 g) infants? *Pediatr Res.* 1991;29:237A

51. Horbar JD, Onstad L, Wright E, NIH Child Health and Human Development Neonatal Research Network. Predicting mortality risk for infants 501–1500 grams at birth: a national institutes of health neonatal research network report. *Crit Care Med.* 1993;21:12–18

52. Paris JJ, Crone RK, Reardon F. Physicians' refusal of treatment: the case of Baby L. *N Engl J Med.* 1990;322:1012–1015

53. Twedt S. Should comatose boy live? Hospital, dad differ. *Pittsburgh Press.* June 3, 1991:1

54. Smothers R. Atlanta court bars efforts to end life support for stricken girl, 13. *New York Times.* October 18, 1991:A10

55. Nelson LJ, Nelson RM. Ethics and the provision of futile, harmful, or burdensome treatment to children. *Crit Care Med.* 1992;20:427–433

56. Truog RD, Brett AS, Frader J. The problem with futility. *N Engl J Med.* 1992;326:1560–1564

57. Storch TG. Passive euthanasia for hypoplastic left heart syndrome. *Am J Dis Child.* 1992;146:1426

58. Armstrong CJ. Judicial involvement in treatment decisions: the emerging consensus. In: Civetta J, Taylor RW, Karby RR, eds. *Critical Care.* Philadelphia, PA: JB Lippincott Co; 1988

# AMERICAN ACADEMY OF PEDIATRICS

# Guidelines for Home Care of Infants, Children, and Adolescents With Chronic Disease

Committee on Children With Disabilities          (RE9530)

Many infants, children, and adolescents with long-term, serious health problems require frequent and/or prolonged hospitalizations that separate them from their home environment. Hospitalization interferes with the ability to form the normal, interpersonal family and community relationships that are important for normal growth and development. Caring for a child at home may be a desirable alternative to hospital-based care.

Caring for a child at home, with all the necessary assistance, is more supportive of the family's traditional caretaking and nurturing role, but home care should be initiated only when consonant with the best interests of the child and family and if adequate resources and support are available. Combining the benefits of home care with appropriate medical treatment and support requires the development of innovative programs among hospitals, physicians, parents, home care professionals, and communities.

Although many home health care programs for patients with chronic disease exist, objective data about their efficiency, risks, benefits, and costs are limited. Where documentation exists,[1,2] home care can be shown to be a successful, cost-effective method of health care delivery. Careful planning and coordination of family, hospital, home care providers, and community resources, however, are essential for successful home health care programs, and guidelines for program development and assessment are needed.

The goal of a home health care program for infants, children, or adolescents with chronic conditions is the provision of comprehensive, cost-effective health care within a nurturing home environment that maximizes the capabilities of the individual and minimizes the effects of the disabilities. This may be established to prevent hospitalization or reduce the length of hospitalization.

## PROGRAM DEVELOPMENT

Comprehensive planning should minimize physical and emotional risk to the patient, adverse effects on the family members, or unforeseen finan-cial burdens. Because of the many factors to be considered, planning should be done by a multidisciplinary Home Health Care Team. This team should include (when available): parents; a primary care pediatrician; other physicians (eg, hospital physicians, subspecialists, other community physicians); nurses; occupational, physical, respiratory, and speech therapists; child development specialists; educational specialists; nutritionists; social workers; teachers; home care providers (eg, home health aide and equipment provider); case managers; and insurers. The team must initially develop the Home Health Care Program, which provides comprehensive care recommendations (the treatment plan) and arrangements based on each individual patient's demonstrated needs (the resources to be utilized, including equipment and service providers). Many of the resources used in the Home Health Care Program may be an extension of existing hospital services.

After the Home Health Care Program is established, each child and family identified for the program needs an Individualized Home Care Plan (IHCP). The family (or other primary caregivers) and the primary care pediatrician must play a major role in developing, implementing, and monitoring the plan, with appropriate subspecialists, when necessary, identified early in this process. A home care service coordinator to support and coordinate the IHCP should be selected (jointly by the team and the family) for each patient. The coordinator, working in conjunction with the primary care pediatrician, works closely with the family, identifying and assisting with their needs in caring for the child at home, including family training about illness, treatment, and advocacy, and assisting families in developing service coordination skills. This family oriented advocate could be an appropriately trained parent of a child with chronic illness who has experience in home care-related issues and concerns. Every effort should be made to identify a single care coordinator for the child and family, even if this requires serving the needs of several programs/systems. If this is not possible, it is essential that a communication system be developed with unique and shared responsibilities delineated for each care coordinator.

## IMPLEMENTATION

### Patient Selection

Eligibility for home health care should be based on a comprehensive analysis of the Home Health Care Program capabilities, whether the child's therapeutic

This statement has been approved by the Council on Child and Adolescent Health.

The recommendations in this statement do not indicate an exclusive course of treatment or procedure to be followed. Variations, taking into account individual circumstances, may be appropriate.

PEDIATRICS (ISSN 0031 4005). Copyright © 1995 by the American Academy of Pediatrics.

needs can be met by home care, the potential benefits and risks, and the available resources. Families should not face excessive pressure to enroll their children in a home care program if this move would be detrimental to the child or family. The patient should participate in the development of the IHCP to the extent possible, with the following factors considered for patient selection.

1. Patient Factors. Underlying any potential for home care in chronic disease is the patient's medical stability vis-à-vis the capacity of the Home Health Care Program to provide backup and emergency care. Previous experience with home care in similar situations should be reviewed. As part of the initial discharge planning process, plans should be made to explore home care as an option to begin when the patient's condition is as stable as possible.
2. Family and Home Factors. If possible, each family should have at least two members trained and fully able to care for the child in the home. In some situations, two or more trained adults are essential to assure medical safety. The family should provide evidence of sufficient parental/family involvement, proven capability in performing medical and nursing tasks, and an appropriate home situation (eg, physical environment, safety, and geographic location) for the child's medical safety to be reasonably assured. Respite services should be part of the plan as well as emergency staffing in case the care provider is ill. Specialized day care should be explored as well.
3. Community Factors. A primary care pediatrician or other provider should be involved in the development of the IHCP before hospital discharge, be knowledgeable about the plan, and agree to participate by providing primary medical care. This physician oversees the medical aspects of the plan after hospital discharge, communicates with the attending physician at the hospital and other involved physicians, and reviews the safety of the plan. The service coordinator must assure the availability of appropriate home health care providers, equipment, and other special needs (eg, oxygen suppliers). Essential equipment must either be portable or available at each site that the child attends. Reasonable contingency plans for emergencies (eg, power and equipment backup for those with life-support devices and appropriate transportation), including clear delineation of the unique and shared medical care responsibilities among physicians on the team, must be available. The "team leader," generally the primary care pediatrician, should be identified.
4. Home Care Trial. In order to identify any omissions or lack of clarity in the IHCP, a successful trial of care by the future home health care providers within the hospital setting (using emergency backup by the regular hospital staff) is recommended before discharge. Family members should use equipment and supplies that will be used at home first in the hospital so that they can become familiar and proficient with their use. Any

differences between hospital use and home use should be addressed before hospital discharge. The trial should enable the family and other regular caregivers to develop self-confidence and avoid overdependency upon hospital staff.

## IHCP DEVELOPMENT

Careful review of the patient's status and needs in the hospital should be made by each professional participating in the patient's care. Each discipline should formulate goals and objectives for the patient and develop daily program components to meet these goals in the home. Thereafter, a meeting should occur to formulate an integrated daily IHCP with specific responsibilities delineated, including the establishment of financial responsibility. This plan includes the following: 1) designation of a home care service coordinator, 2) involvement of a primary care physician who will provide "the medical home," 3) family access to a telephone, 4) specific physician orders for medications, treatments, medical follow-up, and medical tests as appropriate, 5) a plan for monitoring the home care plan that includes designation of the "team leader" and specific responsibilities of the service coordinator and primary care physician, 6) a mechanism for making adjustments to the plan when needed, 7) a defined backup system for medical emergencies, 8) regular or special educational services for school-aged children and early intervention services for eligible infants and toddlers, and 9) criteria procedures for transition from home care, when appropriate.

### Educational Services

Planning for early intervention and/or educational services should stress the importance of educating children in an environment with peers that promotes and maintains socialization. With school systems providing education in the least restrictive environment, the child's Individual Educational Plan should incorporate therapeutic and nursing care that is coordinated with the daily IHCP. A child should not be denied necessary home care services because he or she is entitled to school-based services.

### Equipment and Supplies

Equipment and supplies that are appropriate for use in the home must be selected and secured according to each patient's needs. Community suppliers must guarantee continuous availability, maintenance, emergency repair, and replacement of this equipment. Financial reimbursement to the family for necessary equipment, supplies, and maintenance should not be denied because the care of the patient is transferred from the hospital to the home. Any need for equipment changes, including manufacturer recalls, should be arranged in conjunction with the service coordinator and the family. Equipment performance should be documented and tracked by the manufacturer.

### Child and Caregiver Training

Critical components of the IHCP are education and training for the family and other caregivers, including the child to the greatest extent possible, professional and paraprofessional health care providers, school personnel (if the child will be attending school), and all emergency personnel. Before discharge from the hospital, the family rather than the hospital staff should provide as much of the child's care as possible. The family must learn to recognize and record changes in the child's condition that would require consultation and/or modification of care. The patient, especially if an adolescent, should be encouraged to take responsibility for self-care to the extent appropriate. Although it may require time, restraint, and patience, the hospital staff should assume a supportive, rather than primary, role in this stage of the child's care. The plan should also incorporate outreach education for staff at local hospitals and community-based home care providers.

### Cost

The Home Health Care Team should evaluate the projected cost of the child's IHCP and the available methods of financial support and resolve funding problems before hospital discharge of the patient. There should be continuing review and dialogue among the Home Health Care Team, insurers, and public programs to help assure the financial coverage of home care. Creative financing approaches include negotiated arrangements among a diversity of health care and social service funding sources.

### Effects of Home Care on the Child and the Family

During the development of the child's IHCP, a number of issues related to the potential effects of having a severely ill child at home need to be explored with the family, including issues of privacy, physical burdens of care, impact upon other family members such as siblings, time demands of home care, role of the parents in coordinating care, and the social and financial aspects including issues of confidentiality. Assessment should include impact of home care on family dynamics, activities, and schedules including work-related responsibilities. Discussions with the family should explore possible approaches to these issues before discharge, and the family should feel comfortable with their choices.

## PROGRAM MAINTENANCE

Before discharge and at intervals during the child's home care program, there should be a coordinated review of the patient's and family's needs, how the family is managing, the progress toward the home care goals, and other available relevant information. The service coordinator and the family should conduct the program review, soliciting input from all involved providers. This is particularly important since the child's and family's needs will likely change over time, both medically and socially. The type and frequency of the child's specialized therapy should be reviewed, and any new issues that arise should be evaluated. Home care case management conferences are recommended at periodic intervals. They should include all community-based providers and case managers.

## PROGRAM EVALUATION AND OUTCOME

A review of all patients in the Home Health Care Program and an assessment of data from similar programs should be done by the Home Health Care Team on an ongoing basis. Feedback data for review should be obtained from several sources (eg, the child, the parents, the community, local care providers, and school personnel). Sharing experiences will lead to the continued refinement of the Home Health Care Program. Principles of program review should include the analysis and improvement of key clinical and social outcomes, with evaluation of the ultimate value of the care provided. Follow-up and outcome assessments need to be based on the following: 1) survival, 2) the need for subsequent hospitalizations and other morbidity, 3) developmental progress, 4) course of the underlying disease, 5) actual utilization of resources as compared with expected utilization, 6) financial experience (cash flow and continued availability of benefits), and 7) effects on family members, including siblings. As with all elements of family-centered care, input from family members into this process is essential.

## ALTERNATIVES

The use of intermediate or chronic care facilities may be considered as an alternative to home care. The choice of home care or alternative care must be based upon a thorough evaluation of the needs and wishes of the family and the expected course of the illness. Most effective care planning requires the development of a continuum of care options and the evaluation of alternate types of care. The home is one community-based alternative. Components comprise a spectrum of care that may be required over time depending on changing circumstances.

## CONCLUSION

Home health care programs for infants, children, or adolescents with chronic disease may offer the advantages of supporting the child's growth and development in a more nurturing family environment without compromising comprehensive health care delivered in a cost-effective manner. Since the number of children with chronic diseases that may be appropriate for home care is increasing (eg, technology-dependent children, children with human immunodeficiency virus infection), this issue affects all pediatricians. Careful analysis, shared experience, and future controlled studies will help support the appropriateness and cost-effectiveness of home health care programs in the care of patients with chronic disease. The central role of the family in this process must be recognized and continuously supported, with appropriate ongoing assistance as the needs of the child and family change over time.

COMMITTEE ON CHILDREN WITH DISABILITIES, 1994 TO 1995
James Perrin, MD, Chair
Gerald Erenberg, MD
Robert La Camera, MD
John A. Nackashi, MD
John R. Poncher, MD
Virginia Randall, MD

Renee C. Wachtel, MD
W. Daniel Williamson, MD
Philip R. Ziring, MD

LIAISON REPRESENTATIVES

Polly Arango, Family Voices
Debbie Gaebler, MD, American Academy of Physical
    Medicine and Rehabilitation
Connie Garner, RN, MSN, EdD, US Dept of
    Education Programs
Diane Garro, Social Security Administration
Joseph G. Hollowell, MD, Centers for Disease
    Control and Prevention, Center for Environmental
    Health and Injury Control
John Mather, MD, Social Security Administration
Merle McPherson, MD, Maternal and Child Health
    Bureau, Dept of Health & Human Services

SECTION LIAISON

Harry L. Gewanter, MD, Section on Rheumatology

## REFERENCES

1. Donati MA, Guenette G, Auerbach H. Prospective controlled study of home and hospital therapy of cystic fibrosis pulmonary disease. *J Pediatr.* 1987;111:28–33

2. Frates RC, Splaingard ML, Smith EO, Harrison GM. Outcome of home mechanical ventilation in children. *J Pediatr.* 1985;106:850–856

## SUGGESTED READINGS

Aday LA, Aitken MJ, Wegener DH. *Pediatric Home Care: Results of a National Evaluation of Programs for Ventilator Assisted Children.* Chicago, IL: Pluribus Press; 1988

American Academy of Pediatrics, Committee on Child Health Financing. Health care financing for the child with catastrophic costs. *Pediatrics.* 1987;80:752–757

Burr CK. Impact on the family of a chronically ill child. In: Hobbs N, Perrin JM, eds. *Issues in the Care of Children With Chronic Illness.* San Francisco, CA: Jossey-Bass; 1985:24–40

Feinberg EA. Family stress in pediatric home care. *Caring.* 1985; 4:38–41

Hochstadt NJ, Yost DM, eds. *The Medically Complex Child: The Transition to Home Care.* New York, NY: Harwood Academic Publishers; 1991

Quint R, Chesterman E, Crain LS, Winkleby M, Boyce WT. Home care for ventilator-dependent children: psychosocial impact on the family. *AJDC.* 1990;144:1238–1241

Perrin JM, Shayne MW, Bloom SR. *Home and Community Care for Chronically Ill Children.* New York, NY: Oxford University Press; 1993

Stein RE, ed. *Caring for Children With Chronic Illness.* New York, NY: Springer Publishing Co; 1989

# AMERICAN ACADEMY OF PEDIATRICS

## Health Care of Children in Foster Care   (RE9404)

Committee on Early Childhood, Adoption, and Dependent Care

The foster care system in America has evolved as a means of providing protection and shelter for children who require out-of-home placement.[1] It is designed to be a temporary service, with a goal of either returning children home or arranging for suitable adoptive homes. In recent years, child welfare agencies have been directing greater efforts toward supporting families in crisis to prevent foster care placements whenever feasible and to reunify families as soon as possible when placements cannot be avoided. Increasingly, extended family members are being recruited and assisted in providing kinship care for children when their biologic parents cannot care for them. However, during the past decade the number of children in foster care has nearly doubled, despite landmark federal legislation designed to expedite permanency planning for children in state custody.[2] It is estimated that by 1995 more than 500 000 children will be in foster care.[3] In large part, this unrelenting trend is the result of increased abuse and neglect of children occurring in the context of parental substance abuse, mental illness, homelessness, and human immunodeficiency virus infection.[4] As a result, a disproportionate number of children placed in foster care come from that segment of the population with the fewest social and financial resources and from families that have few personal and limited extended family sources of support.[5]

It is not surprising then that children entering foster care are often in poor health. Compared with children from the same socioeconomic background, they suffer much higher rates of serious emotional and behavioral problems, chronic physical disabilities, birth defects, developmental delays, and poor school achievement.[6-13] Moreover, the health care these children receive while in placement is often compromised by inadequate funding, planning, and coordination of services as well as by poor communication among health and child welfare professionals. Many child welfare agencies lack specific policies for children's physical and mental health services.[14] Despite the broad range of supportive and therapeutic services needed, most children do not undergo a comprehensive developmental or psychological assessment at any time during their placement. State Medicaid systems, which provide funding for the health care of the majority of children in foster care, rarely cover all of the services these children require. Restrictions on covered services, fixed or declining reimbursement to health care providers, increased complexity of billing procedures, and delays in payment of physicians' fees have been linked to a dramatic nationwide decline in the number of physicians participating in state Medicaid programs.[15,16] As a result, many foster parents report difficulty finding health care professionals who are willing to care for these children.[17]

Pediatricians can play a critically important role in helping child welfare agencies, foster families, and biological families to minimize the trauma of placement separation and to improve the child's health and development during the period of foster care. Providing health care to these children requires considerably more time as compared with the time needed by the average pediatric patient. Physicians must be prepared to provide necessary care even when little or no specific information about the child is available at the time of the visit. The pediatrician should attempt to identify physical, psychosocial, and developmental problems and assist social workers and foster parents in determining the types of care and community services the child requires.[18]

This statement builds on a previous Committee statement[19] and provides specific suggestions for delivery of health services to children in foster care placement.

### STANDARDS FOR HEALTH CARE SERVICES

In 1988, the Child Welfare League of America, in consultation with the American Academy of Pediatrics, developed *Standards for Health Care Services for Children in Out-of-Home Care.*[20] This document serves as a comprehensive guideline for developing and organizing health and mental health services for child welfare organizations. Child welfare agencies should be encouraged to adhere to these standards. Pediatricians should become familiar with these standards and assist child welfare administrators, caseworkers, and foster parents in implementing them.

Because children in foster care have a high prevalence of chronic and complex illnesses, establishing continuity of care and ensuring a comprehensive and coordinated treatment approach by all professionals involved in their care should be one of the highest priorities for child welfare agencies. Diverse characteristics of child welfare agencies, wide geographic distribution of foster homes in some states, and lack of comprehensive funding for children's physical and

This statement has been approved by the Council on Child and Adolescent Health.

The recommendations in this statement do not indicate an exclusive course of treatment or serve as a standard of medical care. Variations, taking into account individual circumstances, may be appropriate.

mental health care services contribute to the difficulty of providing an organized approach to the care of these children. To avoid fragmentation of care, a variety of health care delivery models can be developed for this population.

Regardless of the model developed in a locale, it should adhere to certain principles. Whether services are delivered by a single team of professionals under one "roof"[21] or as part of a planned program of care utilizing many different community resources,[10] all professionals involved in the care of each child should communicate effectively with one another. Furthermore, compassionate assistance, education, and training for foster and biologic parents should be included as an integral part of the overall program of services provided to children and their families during and after placement.

Pediatricians should be involved in the planning and development of systems of care for children in foster care. In addition to their role as primary health care providers, pediatricians may be contracted by child welfare agencies to serve as regional and statewide medical consultants and to develop and implement policies and programs that will improve the effectiveness and comprehensiveness of services for children in foster care.[16]

## THE COMPONENTS OF HEALTH CARE SERVICES

Health care services may be divided into four components: initial health screening, comprehensive health assessment, developmental and mental health evaluation, and ongoing monitoring of health status.

### Initial Health Screening

Every child entering foster care should have a health screening evaluation before or shortly after placement. The purpose of this examination is to identify any immediate medical needs the child may have and any additional health conditions of which the foster parents and caseworker should be aware. Careful measurement of height, weight, and head circumference may reveal growth delays and reflect poor nutritional or general health status. Because many children entering foster care have been the victims of physical or sexual abuse, all body surfaces should be unclothed at some point during the physical examination, and any bruises, scars, deformities, or limitations in the function of body parts or organ systems should be noted and recorded. If there is a history of physical abuse before placement, or if signs of recent physical trauma are present, appropriate imaging studies to screen for recent or healing fractures should be considered. Genital and anal examination of both sexes should be conducted and laboratory tests performed for sexually transmitted diseases when indicated clinically or by history. Other infections and communicable diseases, especially pediculosis, should be noted and treated promptly. The status of any known chronic illnesses should be determined to ensure that appropriate medications are available. The physician should discuss specific care instructions directly with the foster parents and not rely on an intermediary.

### Comprehensive Health Assessment

Within 1 month of the child's placement, a comprehensive health assessment should be performed by a pediatrician who is knowledgeable about and interested in the treatment of children in foster care and who can provide regular, ongoing primary care services. Child welfare agencies should make all pertinent past medical, social, and family information available to assist the physician performing the evaluation. Both the child's caseworker and foster parents should be present for the initial visit. Whenever possible, for this and subsequent visits, information should be obtained from the biologic parents, and they should be kept informed about the health status of their child. When appropriate, and as a part of the care plan of the child welfare agency, biologic parents may be encouraged to be present at health care visits and to participate in health care decisions. The historical review should include the circumstances that led to the placement; the child's adjustment to separation from the biologic family; adaptation to the foster home; developmental or school progress; and the agency's plans for a permanent placement (ie, return home, adoption, or long-term foster care). The physical examination should focus on the presence of any acute or chronic medical problems that may require further evaluation or referral. Screening tests should be performed according to the Recommendations for Preventive Pediatric Health Care of the American Academy of Pediatrics.[22] Because many young children entering foster care come from settings in which substance abuse and sexual promiscuity are common, they should be considered to be at high risk for human immunodeficiency virus infection, hepatitis, and other sexually acquired infections. Laboratory tests for these conditions should be performed when appropriate.[23]

Children entering foster care are likely to be incompletely immunized[7] and determining the actual types and number of immunizations that a particular child has received in the past may be difficult. By communicating directly with prior medical providers or reviewing previous medical records, it is often possible to reconstruct the child's immunization history. But, for some children, despite a thorough effort, little or no immunization information will be available. These children should be considered "susceptible" and immunized according to the schedules of the American Academy of Pediatrics.[24,25]

### Developmental and Mental Health Evaluation

At each child health visit, pediatricians should attempt to assess the child's developmental, educational, and emotional status. These assessments may be based on structured interviews with the foster parents and caseworker, the results of standardized tests of development, and/or a review of the child's school progress. All children with identified problems should be further evaluated and treated as clinically indicated. When available, local consultants and community-based intervention programs should be called upon to assist in diagnosing and treating children with developmental and educational problems. Pediatricians may also assist social workers and foster parents by referring eligible children to the various federal and state "entitlement" programs in their community (eg, The Special Supplemental Food Program for Women, Infants and Children; Head Start, Birth-to-Three programs[26]; special education programs[27]; Title V programs).

In some communities, child welfare agencies may be able to access or establish multidisciplinary teams to routinely evaluate children entering foster care. By their very nature, multidisciplinary teams provide both a comprehensive and coordinated approach to assessment and are often an efficient and cost-effective means of accomplishing this task. A successful community-based program model utilizing this approach has been described.[10]

Regardless of how the comprehensive assessment is performed, the results and recommendations should be incorporated into the child's social service case plan. The caseworker and pediatrician should then help the foster parents to arrange for all the services recommended for the child.

### Monitoring of Children's Health Status While in Placement

Placement in foster care is a stressful experience for most children. Often, problems arise during the course of placement that were not apparent at the outset. For example, a child's adjustment to separation from his or her family and adaptation to the foster home may be characterized by distinct behavioral changes over time.[18] Similarly, significant emotional distress may occur after visits with the biologic family members.[28] Therefore, all children in foster care should receive periodic reassessments of their health, development, and emotional status to determine any changes in their status and the need for additional services and interventions. Such reassessments should occur at approximately 6-month intervals in the first year of placement and at least yearly thereafter, depending on the stability of the placement and changes in the child's status. When changes in foster placement are planned, or when decisions regarding permanency planning are anticipated, pediatricians can help child welfare professionals evaluate these decisions in light of the child's age and developmental level. Pediatricians can also work with both the child welfare agency and the court to determine what is truly in the child's "best interests."

### TRANSFER OF MEDICAL INFORMATION

Up to one quarter of children placed in foster care experience three or more changes in foster homes. Furthermore, up to 35% of children reenter the foster care system after being returned to their family. These changes are usually accompanied by changes in health care providers as well.[29] As a result, available health information about these children is often incomplete and spread across many different sites. To enhance continuity of care, several states have developed an abbreviated health record, often called a medical passport.[16] This form is retained by the child's custodian and is designed to facilitate the transfer of essential information among health and mental health professionals. It provides a brief listing of the child's medical problems, allergies, chronic medications, and immunization data, as well as basic social service and family history. Foster parents are instructed to keep this document for the child and to bring it to all health visits. As the child's condition changes, health care providers should update the information on the form. If the child changes foster homes, or returns to his/her biologic family, the medical passport should be transferred too. Computerized health information systems are also being developed in several states that may make specific health information about children in foster care more readily accessible to practitioners and child welfare agencies. However, a foster parent-held medical passport has the potential to play a valuable role in the overall health care of children in foster care for some time to come. Computerized medical records for these children should be accorded the same confidentiality as written records.

### THE IMPACT OF FOSTER CARE PLACEMENT ON CHILDREN

Society has always been reluctant to involuntarily remove children from their parents. Certainly, even brief separation from parental care is an unfortunate and often traumatic event for children.[30] Despite legal mandates to expediently formulate a "permanent plan," many children may remain in foster care interminably while the child welfare and legal systems deliberate their fate. However, concerns about time should be balanced against other evidence that suggests that foster care placement may be a positive and therapeutic intervention for some children. Significant improvements in a child's health status,[9] development, intelligence, school attendance, and academic achievement have been noted consequent to foster care placement.[31] Thus, for children who have suffered severe neglect and abuse, or whose families cannot adequately care for them, placement in foster care can be a significant opportunity to receive important intervention and rehabilitation and should not be considered only as an option of last resort.

### RECOMMENDATIONS

1. Pediatricians should participate in the care of children in foster care as primary health care providers and as consultants to child welfare agencies. Child welfare agencies and pediatricians should work together to implement the standards for health care of children in foster care developed by the Child Welfare League of America and the American Academy of Pediatrics.
2. All children entering foster care should have an initial physical examination before or soon after placement. This examination should focus on identifying acute and chronic conditions requiring expedient treatment.
3. All children in foster care should receive comprehensive physical and mental health evaluations within 1 month of placement. Pediatricians and child welfare agencies should work together to ensure that children in foster care receive the full range of therapeutic services needed and partici-

pate in all federal and state entitlement programs for which they are eligible.

4. While in placement, the child's physical and mental health status and progress should be monitored at least twice a year in the first year of placement and at least yearly thereafter. However, more frequent reassessment may be indicated based on the child's age, change in foster home, or change in physical or mental health status. Individual social service case plans should include the results and incorporate the recommendations of health professionals.

5. Child welfare agencies should develop and implement systems to ensure the efficient transfer of medical and mental health information among professionals who treat children in foster care.

COMMITTEE ON EARLY CHILDHOOD, ADOPTION, AND DEPENDENT CARE, 1993 to 1994
Edward L. Schor, MD, Chair
Charles G. Erickson, MD
Barbara J. M. Evans, MD
Sherrel L. Hammar, MD
Susan A. Keathley, MD
Peter M. Miller, MD
Jody R. Murph, MD
Mark D. Simms, MD, MPH

LIAISON REPRESENTATIVES
The Honorable Julie A. Edwards, National Council of Juvenile and Family Court Judges
Eileen Mayers Pasztor, DSW, Child Welfare League of America
Marilyn Smith, National Association for the Education of Young Children
Phyllis Stubbs, MD, Head Start Health Services Program
Susan Weber, Special Assistant to the Commissioner, Administration on Children, Youth, and Families

AAP SECTION LIAISON
Daniel Bronfin, MD, Section on Community Pediatrics
Carol Roberts Gerson, MD, Section on Otolaryngology

## REFERENCES

1. Simms MD. Foster children and the foster care system, I: history and legal structure. *Curr Probl Pediatr.* 1991;21:297–321
2. Publ L No. 96–272. *The Adoption Assistance Child Welfare Act of 1980.* Washington, DC: Government Printing Office; 1980
3. US House of Representatives, Select Committee on Children, Youth, Families. *No Place to Call Home: Discarded Children in America.* Washington, DC: US Government Printing Office; 1989
4. National Commission on Family Foster Care. *A Blueprint for Fostering Infants, Children, and Youths in the 1990s.* Washington, DC: Child Welfare League of America; 1991
5. Tomlinson P. *Child Welfare Statistical Fact Book.* McLean, VA: Maximus; 1984
6. Frank G. Treatment needs of children in foster care. *Am J Orthopsychiatry.* 1980;50:256–263
7. Schor EL. The foster care system and health status of foster children. *Pediatrics.* 1982;69:521–528
8. Moffatt ME, Peddie M, Stulginskas J, Pless IB, Steinmetz N. Health care delivery to foster children: a study. *Health Soc Work.* 1985;10:129–137
9. White R, Benedict MI. Health status and utilization patterns of children in foster care: executive summary. Washington, DC: US Department of Health and Human Services, Administration for Children, Youth, and Families; 1986. Grant No. 90-PD-86509
10. Simms MD. The foster care clinic: a community program to identify treatment needs of children in foster care. *J Dev Behav Pediatr.* 1989;10: 121–128
11. Kavaler F, Swire MR. *Foster Child Health Care.* Lexington, MA: Lexington Books; 1983
12. Dubowitz H, Feigelman S, Zuravin S, Tepper V, Davidson N. The physical health of children in kinship care. *AJDC.* 1992;146:603–610
13. Halfon N, Berkowitz G, Klee L. Children in foster care in California: an examination of Medicaid reimbursed health services utilization. *Pediatrics.* 1992;89:1230–1237
14. Schor EL. Health care supervision of foster children. *Child Welfare.* 1981; 60:313–319
15. Yudkowsky BK, Cartland JD, Flint SS. Pediatrician participation in Medicaid: 1978 to 1989. *Pediatrics.* 1990;85:567–577
16. Simms MD, Kelly RW. Pediatricians and foster children. *Child Welfare.* 1991;70:451–461
17. Halfon N, Klee L. Health and development services for children with multiple needs: the child in foster care. *Yale Law and Policy Rev.* 1991;9: 71–96
18. Simms MD. Foster children and the foster care system, II: impact on the child. *Curr Probl Pediatr.* 1991;21:345–369
19. American Academy of Pediatrics, Committee on Early Childhood, Adoption, Dependent Care. Health care of foster children. *Pediatrics.* 1987;79:644–646
20. Child Welfare League of America. *Standards for Health Care Services for Children in Out-of-Home Care.* Washington, DC: Child Welfare League of America; 1988
21. Schor EL, Neff JM, LaAsmar JL. The Chesapeake Health Plan: an HMO model for foster children. *Child Welfare.* 1984;63:431–440
22. American Academy of Pediatrics, Committee on Psychosocial Aspects of Child and Family Health. *Guidelines for Health Supervision II.* Elk Grove Village, IL: American Academy of Pediatrics; 1988:155–159
23. American Academy of Pediatrics, Task Force on Pediatric AIDS. Infants and children with acquired immunodeficiency syndrome: placement in adoption and foster care. *Pediatrics.* 1989;83:609–612
24. American Academy of Pediatrics, Committee on Infectious Diseases. *Report of the Committee on Infectious Diseases.* 22nd ed. Elk Grove Village, IL: American Academy of Pediatrics; 1991:18
25. American Academy of Pediatrics, Committee on Infectious Diseases. Universal hepatitis B immunization. *Pediatrics.* 1992;89:795–800
26. Publ L No. 99–457. *Education of the Handicapped Amendments of 1986.* Washington, DC: Government Printing Office; 1986
27. Publ L No. 94–142. *Education for All Handicapped Children Act of 1975.* Washington, DC: Government Printing Office; 1975
28. Gean MP, Gillmore JL, Dowler JK. Infants and toddlers in supervised custody: a pilot study of visitation. *J Am Acad Child Psychiatry.* 1985;24: 608–612
29. Schor EL. Foster care. *Pediatr Clin North Am.* 1988;35:1241–1252
30. Littner N. *Some Traumatic Effects of Separation Placement.* New York, NY: Child Welfare League of America; 1976
31. Fanshel D, Shinn EB. *Children in Foster Care: A Longitudinal Investigation.* New York, NY: Columbia University Press; 1978

# AMERICAN ACADEMY OF PEDIATRICS

## Health Needs of Homeless Children and Families     (RE9637)

Committee on Community Health Services

**ABSTRACT.** The intent of this statement is to substantiate the existence of homelessness in virtually every community, illustrate the pervasive health and psychosocial problems facing the growing population of children who are homeless, and encourage practitioners to include homeless children in their health care delivery practices, social services, and advocacy efforts. The recommendations will guide practitioners in taking actions to diminish the severe negative impact that living in temporary shelters has on the health and well-being of developing children. In this statement the American Academy of Pediatrics reaffirms its stance that homeless children need permanent dwellings in order to thrive.

An increasing number of children and families in virtually all communities in the United States are either homeless or living in tenuous situations that put them at a profoundly high risk of losing their homes, a most basic human necessity.

Families with children are the fastest growing subgroup of the homeless population nationally and represent more than half of the homeless population in many cities.[1] Lack of a permanent dwelling deprives children of one of the most basic necessities for proper growth and development and poses unique risks for homeless children that compromise their health status. Pediatricians are encouraged to be aware of this growing population of children and include them in their health care delivery practices, social services, and advocacy efforts.

### BACKGROUND

The term homeless, as defined by the Department of Housing and Urban Development (HUD), includes those who are homeless, ie, living on the streets or in shelters, and those who are at risk of being homeless. Included in the latter group are those who find themselves in: 1) precarious arrangements attempting to stay in conventional housing, including the increasing number of children living in poverty or in single-parent families, those who are recent immigrants, and those caught in the complicated web of urban decay and conflicting housing and social policies; 2) the process of termination of a stay in an institutional setting; or 3) situations in which they have insufficient prospects or resources.[2]

Each year an estimated 2.5 to 3 million people lack access to a conventional dwelling or residence, and it is estimated that families with children account for up to 43% of the homeless population.[1,3,4] Although there is disagreement concerning the exact number of homeless persons, there is consensus that the numbers are large and continuing to grow. In 1994, requests for emergency shelter increased in 30 major cities by an average of 13%, with 9 of 10 of the cities reporting an increase in requests from families.[4] In 87% of those cities, emergency shelters may have to turn away homeless families with children because of limited resources; 73% of the surveyed cities identified homeless families with children as a group for whom shelter and other services were particularly lacking.[4] There were 1900 shelters counted by HUD in 1984; by 1988, there were 5400 shelters. In 1984, 21% of the homeless requiring emergency shelter were families; that percentage increased to 40% in 1988.[5]

Several societal problems contribute to the increasing rate of homelessness among American families, including lack of affordable housing; decreases in availability of rent subsidies; unemployment, especially among those who have held only marginal jobs; personal crises such as divorce and domestic violence; cutbacks in public welfare programs; substance abuse; deinstitutionalization of the mentally ill; and increasing rates of poverty. Although traditionally the homeless population has predominantly been made up of single adults, today families with children account for up to 43% of the homeless population. In some cities, children account for an average of 60% of homeless family members (eg, San Antonio, TX; St Louis, MO; Minneapolis, MN; and Kansas City, MO), and in New York, NY, and Trenton, NJ, children are estimated to account for as much as 75% of homeless family members.[3] Of the 30 cities surveyed by the US Conference of Mayors, 27 (90%) reported increases of families with children among the homeless population.[4]

Most homeless children are temporarily housed with their families in shelters and missions operated by religious organizations and public agencies. However, in many cities, public agencies contract with private hotels to provide temporary housing to homeless people. A 1990 study of public shelter use in New York, NY, and Philadelphia, PA, showed a disproportionate impact of homelessness on minorities, especially black families. In both cities about 7% of black children had spent time in a public shelter between 1990 and 1992, in contrast to less than 1% of white children.[1(p38)]

Whereas maternal education is a potent predictor of children's poverty in the United States, and home-

---

PEDIATRICS (ISSN 0031 4005). Copyright © 1996 by the American Academy of Pediatrics.

less children are far more likely to be impoverished, the link between maternal education and homelessness is not clear. Fifty-three percent of homeless families are headed by young, single women, the majority of whom have graduated from high school or finished some college.[6] In one study, 89% of homeless mothers had been physically or sexually abused, 67% during childhood. A significant percentage had also abused alcohol or drugs.[5]

In addition to those homeless adolescents who are with their families, by conservative estimates, there are also 100 000 to 300 000 adolescents who are living on the streets without supervision, support, or guidance.[7] There are myriad reasons why these youth leave home, including serious conflicts with parents, dysfunctional families, physical and sexual abuse, and neglect.

## HEALTH AND OTHER PROBLEMS ASSOCIATED WITH HOMELESSNESS

Common acute problems in homeless children include upper respiratory tract infections, scabies, lice, tooth decay, ear infections, skin infections, diaper rash, and conjunctivitis.[5] In addition, the incidence of trauma-related injuries, developmental delays, and chronic disease, eg, sinusitis, anemia, asthma, bowel dysfunction, eczema, visual deficits, and neurologic deficits is notably higher for homeless children than for others.[5]

In a Los Angeles study, it was found that homeless families were more likely to use emergency services for preventive and sick care than were domiciled poor families. Moreover, access to care is a formidable barrier for such families.[8]

It is estimated that 30% to 50% of the nation's 220 000 to 280 000 school-age homeless children do not attend school. Of those in school, sporadic attendance, grade repetition, and below-average performance (designated as having special needs) are common.[9] The rate of developmental problems is two to three times higher in homeless children than in poor children who are not homeless.[10]

Although iron deficiency anemia is found to be two to three times more common in homeless children than in children who are not homeless, the most prevalent nutritional problem appears to be obesity.[11] Since refrigeration storage and cooking facilities are not available, fast-food restaurants and convenience stores are often the most common sources for food for homeless individuals. As a result, their diets often contain an excessive amount of carbohydrates and fats. Hunger is another common problem, with a significant number of homeless children lacking sufficient caloric intake.

Access to health care, particularly preventive health care, is impaired for homeless families. Health becomes a lower priority as parents struggle to meet the family's daily demands for food and shelter. Families are so often relocating that there is no opportunity to develop an ongoing relationship with a health care provider. When there is an acute problem, hospital emergency rooms, visiting public health nurses, and clinics usually are relied on to provide episodic and fragmented care. Continuity of care is nonexistent and care is rarely comprehensive, resulting in high rates of underimmunization and other unmet health needs.

Living in a shelter not only separates families from their usual sources of support in the community but also imposes severe hardships in carrying out daily sustenance activities. Despite the fact that families with children are the fastest growing segment of the homeless population, 53% of shelters in 30 major surveyed cities often cannot house families together.[4] Rarely are homeless families housed in their originating neighborhoods. Schooling for children is therefore interrupted and often the family is separated from social networks and institutional support systems, such as day care and health care. Within temporary living situations, refrigeration storage, cooking facilities, opportunities for privacy, bathrooms, quiet quarters for reading and studying, storage space, telephones, and appropriate bedding may be unavailable. Sanitation, safety, and stability are often lacking.[9] These impediments create unique health and social problems for homeless children.

Because young people living on the street often resort to "survival" sex (exchanging sexual activity for shelter, food, protection, or drugs), they are at significant risk of HIV infection, as well as other sexually transmitted diseases. Moreover, the incidence of pregnancy, alcohol and drug abuse, mental illness, and poor nutrition in this population is very high.

## RECOMMENDATIONS

The American Academy of Pediatrics recognizes the severe negative impact that living in temporary shelters can have on the health and well-being of a developing child. The Academy recommends the following actions:

1. Pediatricians should be aware that homelessness is a pervasive societal problem and that children need permanent dwellings. They should be knowledgeable about the existence of homelessness in their own communities and are encouraged to become involved in local relief and advocacy programs. Pediatricians need to be supportive of collaborative efforts on behalf of homeless children.
2. Pediatricians should be involved in the development of national guidelines regarding health and safety standards for temporary residences that house children and families that can be distributed to all states, local governments, and agencies involved with issues of homelessness.
3. Pediatricians should educate social service agencies about the medical problems for which homeless children are at risk, and they should work with these agencies to develop comprehensive systems of care and to strive to ensure that every homeless child and family has a medical home.[12]
4. Comprehensive and coordinated services should be integral to all efforts on behalf of homeless children and families; this is especially critical for children with chronic illnesses and mental health problems.

5. Pediatricians should encourage federal, state, and local governments to support and provide adequate funding for comprehensive homeless prevention programs (including mental health and dental care) to ensure a continuum of care for homeless children and their families.

6. Pediatricians should encourage federal, state, and local governments to appropriate sufficient monies to fund primary health care grants for the provision of comprehensive health care for all homeless people, with a focus on continuity of preventive care.

7. Pediatricians should encourage Congress to fund additional mental health grants for community-based organizations that serve homeless children.

8. As welfare and health care reform move forward, pediatricians should ensure that monitoring systems be devised that will track potentially untoward, as well as positive, effects of these reform initiatives.

COMMITTEE ON COMMUNITY HEALTH SERVICES, 1995 TO 1996
Michael Weitzman, MD, Chair
Stanley I. Fisch, MD
Robert E. Holmberg, Jr, MD
Rudolph E. Jackson, MD
Arthur D. Lisbin, MD
Carolyn J. McKay, MD
Paul Melinkovich, MD
R. Larry Meuli, MD, MPH
Yvette L. Piovanetti, MD

LIAISON REPRESENTATIVES
Anne E. Dyson, MD
  AAP Partnership for Children
Lindsey K. Grossman, MD
  Section on Community and International Child Health
Jennie A. McLaurin, MD, MPH
  Migrant Clinicians Network
Charles Poland III, DDS
  American Academy of Pediatric Dentistry
Janet S. Schultz, MA, CRNP
  National Association of Pediatric Nurse Associates and Practitioners

CONSULTANTS
Michelle S. Jones, MD
Donna O'Hare, MD

## REFERENCES

1. Children's Defense Fund. *The State of America's Children Yearbook*. Washington, DC: Children's Defense Fund; 1994:37–44
2. Burt M. *Alternative Methods to Estimate the Number of Homeless Children and Youth*. Washington, DC: The Urban Institute; 1992
3. Weinreb L, Bassuk E. Health care of homeless families: a growing challenge for family medicine. *J Fam Pract*. 1990;31:74–80
4. US Conference of Mayors. *A Status Report on Hunger and Homelessness in America's Cities: 1994*. Washington, DC: US Conference of Mayors; 1994
5. Bassuk E. Homeless families. *Scientific American*. 1991;December:66–74
6. Wood D. Homeless children: their evaluation and treatment. *J Pediatr Health Care*. 1989;3:194–199
7. Bucy J, Nichols N. Homeless youth: statement of problem and suggested policies. *J Health Social Policy*. 1991;2:65–71
8. Wood D. Barriers to medical care for homeless families compared with housed poor families. *Am J Dis Child*. 1991;145:1109–1115
9. Bassuk E, Rubin L. Homeless children: a neglected population. *Am J Orthopsychiatry*. 1987;57:279–286
10. Bassuk EL, Rubin L, Lauriat AS. Characteristics of sheltered homeless families. *Am J Public Health*. 1986;76:1097–1101
11. Wright J. Children in and of the streets. *Am J Dis Child*. 1991;145:516–519
12. American Academy of Pediatrics, Ad Hoc Task Force on Definition of the Medical Home. The medical home. *Pediatrics*. 1992;90:774

# AMERICAN ACADEMY OF PEDIATRICS

## Pediatric Services for Infants and Children With Special Health Care Needs (RE9318)

Committee on Children With Disabilities

The discipline of infant and child development has expanded greatly during the last 3 decades.[1] Much of this growth is due to new knowledge regarding special services that can improve early development of children with, or at risk for, disabilities.[2] Passage of Public Law 101-476, the Individuals With Disabilities Education Act (IDEA) revising Public Law 99-457,[3] particularly Part H, coupled with existing federal child care mandates and increasing public expression of concern regarding all forms of child care, shows a significant national commitment to the concept that early services are critical if children with disabilities are to reach their full potential.[4]

While there may be debate over the relative importance of environmental vs hereditary factors in a child's developmental outcome, any approach used to promote child development must consider how these factors interact. A child's intelligence, temperament, and motor skills combine in a complex fashion with family and peers, to influence his or her development. There is much to learn about how to positively influence child/caregiver/societal interactions. As work in the area of early intervention* grows, attempts to prove that such efforts can help a child with disabilities overcome innate cognitive and motor skill limitations have met with inconsistent and often controversial results.[5] Improved outcomes are most likely to occur when services are based on the premise that parents or primary caregivers are the most important factors influencing a child's development. All services, even those as clear-cut as a specific health intervention, must follow this premise.[6–8]

Future studies documenting successful outcomes of programs influencing child development—namely measures of effects on cognitive and motor development—need to be expanded to include at least the following variables:

- the child's acceptance into the family
- the child's interpersonal skills
- stabilization of rather than "curing" health problems
- building capacities, even within the context of significant limitations, to maximize the potential for independence and productivity in adult life.

Because of a growing awareness that the family is the most important influence for the child with a developmental disability, research in early intervention increasingly has focused on understanding the family environment. The availability of one or two parents, the family's socioeconomic status, family members' mental and physical health status, and parental intelligence and knowledge of the basics of child care and development are among the important factors that should be considered when evaluating those services that a child may need. Families of children with "special needs" are also becoming strong advocates for participation in the planning of services for their children. As the family's role expands, methods of measuring the effectiveness of early services must increasingly relate not only to specific outcomes for the child, but also to the family's adaptation to the child's disability, to improvement in the family's coping abilities, and to the general strength of the family unit. As services focus increasingly on family models, they must move from the traditional curing model to one of coping, stabilization, and constructive adaptation.

Resources for young children with special health care needs include social, educational, and health services delivered through a variety of agencies, preschool facilities, medical and other health programs. Eligibility criteria for these programs can include such factors as family socioeconomic status or the child's disability. Under the provisions of IDEA, Part H, individual states retain the right to determine eligibility criteria for services funded by this legislation. Funding for these services comes from a number of different sources.

The emphasis in all services for disabled individuals, including those in the very young age groups, should be focused on integrating the child into appropriate community supports as well as health care services used by all children and their families. An important challenge for those developing the health care portion of early intervention services for children with disabilities is to develop a system that responds both to the generic and specialized health

This statement has been approved by the Council on Child and Adolescent Health.

The recommendations in this policy statement do not indicate an exclusive course of treatment or serve as a standard of medical care. Variations, taking into account individual circumstances, may be appropriate.

Received for publication Mar 15, 1993; accepted Mar 15, 1993.

PEDIATRICS (ISSN 0031 4005). Copyright © 1993 by the American Academy of Pediatrics.

* Early intervention services are health, educational, and psychosocial services made available to infants and toddlers with or at risk for disabilities and for their families. These services are based on a written plan of management determined by an interdisciplinary team including a pediatrician or their designee that has appropriately assessed the strengths and needs of the child and family.

care needs of these children in a way that provides expert and appropriate care while respecting the principles of normalization and community integration.

Pediatricians frequently are asked to support or prescribe therapeutic interventions, such as physical and occupational therapy, for infants and children with significant functional limitations. Although objective guidelines are not currently available, it is clear that therapy prescriptions should be written only to facilitate specific needs, be frequently reviewed, and be renewed only if there is indication that the therapy is accomplishing its intended purpose.

The American Academy of Pediatrics supports the belief that the planning and delivery of health care services to children with disabilities at the community, state, and national levels should include, at a minimum, the following principles.

1. Every infant, including those with disabilities or at risk to have a disability, should:

   * be born to parents who have access to information and services that allow their infant the best opportunity to be free of inherited and acquired disease or disability;
   * be born in settings that support the process of immediate parent-child interaction and provide access to ongoing parenting education;
   * have access to immediate emergency care for life-threatening or high-risk conditions;
   * have access to programs that identify, ameliorate, or cure when possible, disease states or conditions that might compromise health and development;
   * have parental access to programs designed to enhance their ability to nurture the child physically and emotionally; and
   * receive perinatal care in a system that shares parent and child information with practitioners and public systems providing ongoing health care supervision and monitoring of developmental risk factors during the developmental period.

2. In addition to services required by every infant, every infant or toddler suspected of having a disability should receive care in a system that:

   * recognizes the need for the early detection and treatment or correction of health disorders, including problems associated with feeding, sleeping, elimination, and temperament; and the identification of conditions with a high probability of causing developmental delay;
   * provides for the timely detection of sensory, cognitive, and emotional disorders;
   * assists families in identifying their child's developmental strengths and needs;
   * develops and monitors a written plan of service addressing child and family needs determined by early interdisciplinary evaluations, including an appropriate medical component;

   * develops a plan of required services without primary concern for the mechanism of payment;
   * coordinates the plan of services with the professionals most involved at any one time in the child's development;
   * includes in the plan the requirement for at least annual reevaluation by appropriately qualified medical personnel in order to determine continuation or change in services;
   * respects the parents' key role in the child's development, and their right to participate in decisions affecting their child and family;
   * provides parents with information and support upon suspicion or diagnosis of developmental delay or disability;
   * encourages and promotes the family's right to participate in the development and coordination of the individualized service plan or equivalent, to the full extent of its desire and ability;
   * coordinates the delivery of services with local agencies and other community health providers, including access to necessary pediatric subspecialty services; and
   * promotes and develops appropriate, community-wide services for the prevention of disabilities.

Pediatricians providing clinical services to infants or toddlers, as well as all others involved in planning, funding, or approving such services at the community, state, or national level, should be familiar with the previously stated principles of care. Parents depend on physicians to routinely monitor their child's development and physical and emotional growth and to inform them when deviations are detected and corrective actions required. Only with appropriate physician surveillance can parents be assured that needed early intervention services will be initiated at appropriate times. In addition, parents can be assured that their child's entitlement to the provisions included in IDEA, Public Law 101-476, will be protected only if physicians recognize the need for their personal involvement in the planning, implementation, and monitoring of all health-related early intervention services.

The American Academy of Pediatrics encourages pediatricians to learn about the developmental needs of children with special needs in order to participate in early intervention.[8] This knowledge, coupled with an understanding of the principles previously presented, can serve to strengthen working relationships with the child's family and involved child care professionals which will benefit the child.

Committee on Children With Disabilities, 1992 to 1993
James Perrin, MD, Chair
Gerald Erenberg, MD
Ruth K. Kaminer, MD
Robert La Camera, MD
John A. Nackashi, MD
John R. Poncher, MD
Virginia Randall, MD
Renee C. Wachtel, MD
Philip R. Ziring, MD

Liaison Representatives
Connie Garner, RN, MSN, EdD, US Dept of
   Education Programs
Ross Hays, MD, American Academy of Physical
   Medicine and Rehabilitation
Joseph G. Hollowell, MD, Centers for Disease
   Control and Prevention, Center for
   Environmental Health and Injury Control

Section Liaison
Harry Gewanter, MD, Section on Rheumatology

Consultant
Alfred Healy, MD

## REFERENCES

1. Kagan J. Overview: perspectives on human infancy. In: Osofsky JD, ed. *Handbook of Infant Development*. New York, NY: John Wiley & Sons; 1979:1–25
2. The Infant Health Development Program. Enhancing the outcomes of low birthweight, premature infants: a multi-site, randomized trial. *JAMA*. 1990;263:3035–3042
3. The Education of the Handicapped Act Amendments of 1986. Section 619
4. Social Security Act, 42 USC 701, Title V, Section 501. Omnibus Budget Reconciliation Act of 1989. Public Law 101-386
5. Bryant DM, Ramey CT. An analysis of the effectiveness of early intervention programs for environmentally at-risk children. In: Guralnick MJ, Bennett FC, eds. *The Effectiveness of Early Intervention for At-Risk and Handicapped Children*. San Diego, CA: Academic Press; 1987:33–75
6. Gartner A, Lipsky DK, Turnbull A. *Supporting Families With a Child With a Disability: An International Outlook*. Baltimore, MD: Paul H. Brookes Publishing; 1991:73–78
7. Shelton TL, Jeppson ES, Johnson BH. *Family Centered Care for Children With Special Health Needs*. Washington, DC: Association for the Care of Children's Health; 1987
8. American Academy of Pediatrics, Maternal Child Health Bureau. *Proceedings From a National Conference on Public Law 99-457: Physician Participation in the Implementation of the Law*. Elk Grove Village, IL: American Academy of Pediatrics; November 1988

# AMERICAN ACADEMY OF PEDIATRICS

## Pediatrician's Role in the Development and Implementation of an Individual Education Plan (IEP) and/or an Individual Family Service Plan (IFSP)    (RE9242)

Committee on Children With Disabilities

Approximately 10% of young persons between the ages of 6 and 17 years receive special education and related services.[1] An additional 750 000 neonates each year may have or be at risk for having developmental disabilities.[2] Therefore, pediatricians have many patients who have disabling conditions or are at risk for them.

Federal legislation requires each child identified as having a disability to have a written plan of service: an Individual Education Plan (IEP) for children aged 3 through 21 years or an Individual Family Service Plan (IFSP) for children aged birth through 2 years. The pediatrician is in a unique position to be involved in planning and providing care for both groups of children.

### BACKGROUND

#### The Individual Education Plan

In 1975 Congress passed Public Law 94-142, the Education for All Handicapped Children Act, as an educational bill of rights to guarantee handicapped children a free and appropriate education. The law required that identification, diagnosis, education, and related services be provided for children 5 to 18 years of age. In 1977, the age range was extended to include children aged 3 to 21 years, with services for children aged 3 to 5 years remaining optional. Not only were these services to be provided, but states also were encouraged to seek out children who had not been served previously.

Conditions eligible under Public Law 94-142 include mental retardation, hearing deficiencies, speech and language impairments, specific learning disabilities, visual handicaps, emotional disturbances, orthopedic impairments, and a variety of other medical conditions categorized as "other health impaired." To be eligible for service under the legislation, a child must have an identifiable condition that has the potential to interfere with his or her educational process and normal school performance to the extent that special education services are required.

Other components of the legislation include the following provisions. (1) Each child must be evaluated by a multidisciplinary team. This team is responsible for designing an IEP that contains specific educational and therapeutic strategies and goals. All such plans are reviewed annually. (2) Each child must be educated in the least restrictive environment or with nonhandicapped students to the greatest extent possible. This criterion supports the concept of integration. (3) Related services, such as transportation, speech pathology, audiology, counseling, physical therapy, and medical services (for diagnosis only), shall be provided when deemed necessary by the evaluating team. (4) The parents' and the child's rights to "due process" shall be protected. This ensures the parents' right to be involved in educational decisions and to obtain redress through an appropriate hearing process when the team's decision is viewed as inappropriate or harmful. A 1987 American Academy of Pediatrics statement encouraged pediatricians to be aware of and partake in the process of formulating an IEP, reviewing it with parents, providing counsel, and coordinating the educational program with the medical treatment plan.[3]

#### The Individual Family Service Plan

In 1986 Congress enacted the Education of the Handicapped Act Amendments, Public Law 99-457.[4] The statute calls for "a statewide, comprehensive, coordinated, multidisciplinary, interagency program of early intervention services for all handicapped infants and their families." The bill does not mandate services but does strengthen incentives. Almost all states have established a program for children aged birth through 3 years. These services are specified as "developmental services . . . to meet a handicapped infant's or toddler's developmental needs in any one or more of the following areas: physical development; cognitive development; speech and language development; psycho-social development; or self-help skills." The purpose of these services is to enhance the development of handicapped infants and toddlers to minimize their potential for developmental delay. It also should reduce education costs to the public schools by minimizing the need for special education services after the youngsters reach school age, minimize the need for institutionalization, enhance the potential for independent living, and the families' abilities to meet special needs.

This statement has been approved by the Council on Child and Adolescent Health.
PEDIATRICS (ISSN 0031 4005). Copyright © 1992 by the American Academy of Pediatrics.

The law requires that each state create its own definition of developmental delay as a basis for determining eligibility for services. The pediatrician has a significant role in determining this eligibility by advocating for a broad definition of developmental delay. If states participate, services must be provided for children already experiencing developmental delay as well as for those diagnosed with a condition that has a high probability of causing delay. In addition, states may elect to provide services to those children who are at risk of manifesting developmental disabilities at a later time.

A major difference between Public Laws 99-457 and 92-142 is that Public Law 99-457 focuses on the family. Under this law, the evaluation, assessment, and planning take place with full family participation and approval.

Children identified as "at risk" receive a comprehensive multidisciplinary assessment. The assessment describes the abilities and needs of the child and family. Following assessment, an IFSP is created. IFSP elements include statements on the following:

1. the child's present attainments
2. family strengths
3. how to enhance development of handicapped infants and toddlers
4. major outcomes expected, including criteria, procedures, and time lines to achieve specific goals
5. specific early intervention services that will help the child and family
6. projected dates for initiating services and their duration
7. name of the case manager responsible for helping the family implement and coordinate the plan
8. steps to help the child and family with the transition to school services at an appropriate time.

The statute specifies a wide array of other services, but the only health services included are those that are "necessary for the infant or toddler to benefit from other early intervention services." Diagnostic and consultative medical services may also be provided.

## MEDICAL ROLE AND RECOMMENDATIONS

There are several roles for the pediatrician under Public Laws 94-142 and 99-457.[5] Not every pediatrician will be comfortable being engaged fully in each role. However, all pediatricians should ensure that every handicapped child in their practice has access to the following services:

1. Conventional health care.
2. Screening and surveillance. The pediatrician should screen all children from the first encounter checking for risk of a handicapping condition or developmental delay. Pediatricians are in key positions to identify at the earliest possible age those children who may benefit from services under Public Laws 94-142 and 99-457. Pediatricians should provide screening and surveil-

lance using a combination of methods best designed to take advantage of multiple sources of information.
3. Participation in assessment. A child identified through screening or observation as being "at risk" for developmental delay should receive a comprehensive multidisciplinary assessment. The pediatrician has an important role as a referral source or, if more extensive participation is elected, as a member of a multidisciplinary team. Not all pediatricians may be comfortable participating in an in-depth assessment. However, all pediatricians should remain in communication with the assessment team.
4. Counsel and advice. During the assessment process, families will need a knowledgeable source of medical advice and counsel. Most assessment teams nominate a member as case manager to work with families. There should be a strong link between the assessment team and the primary care pediatrician and an open sharing of concerns between parents, the pediatrician, and the assessment team.
5. Creating the IEP and IFSP. Pediatricians who participate in the assessment process should be consulted when these documents are created. The assessment team and pediatrician can consult via various routes of communication, ie, in person, by telephone, or by mail. Such consultation is vital to preparing an appropriate and effective plan. When the pediatrician does not serve on the assessment team, he or she should review the plan developed, counsel the family, and prepare to comment as needed. The pediatrician should determine if the health-related services proposed are appropriate and sufficiently comprehensive. He/she should assist parents in performing their advocacy tasks when there is evidence of inappropriate planning. Ideally, when schools or educational agencies are involved in developing the IEP or IFSP, a pediatrician should serve as a member of the assessment team.
6. Coordinated medical services. When health services are part of the IEP or IFSP, they should be carried out by the primary care pediatrician or an appropriate subspecialist. Services and communication should be coordinated in those cases where the patients have complex medical needs involving several physicians or centers.
7. Advocacy. Pediatricians have many local and state opportunities to serve as knowledgeable and thoughtful advocates for improved community services for handicapped children. Pediatricians who select this role need to be aware of the structure of services in the community and the key persons who implement them.

## CONCLUSION

Only by participating in interdisciplinary efforts for children with disabilities can the pediatrician focus on the needs of the whole child and improve the coordination of all forms of service and care.

COMMITTEE ON CHILDREN WITH DISABILITIES, 1991 to 1992
Alfred Healy, MD, Chairman
Gerald Erenberg, MD
Robert La Camera, MD
Ruth K. Kaminer, MD
John A. Nackashi, MD
John Poncher, MD
Virginia F. Randall, MD
Renee C. Wachtel, MD
Philip R. Ziring, MD

Liaison Representatives
Connie Garner, RN, MSN, EdD, US Department of Education Programs
Ross Hays, MD, American Academy of Physical Medicine and Rehabilitation
Joseph G. Hollowell, MD, Centers for Disease Control and Center for Environmental Health and Injury Control

Jeri Nelson, MD, Association for Retarded Citizens of America

Section Liaison
Harry Gewanter, MD, Section on Rheumatology

Consultant
Julian S. Haber

## REFERENCES

1. 12th Annual Report to Congress on Implementation of Handicapped Act. Washington, DC: US Dept of Education, Office of Special Education Programs; 1990:45
2. Haber JS. A four stage approach to early childhood intervention. *Educational Resources.* Champaign, IL: University of Illinois Press; 1989
3. American Academy of Pediatrics, Committee on Children with Disabilities. Pediatrician's role in development and implementation of an individual education plan. *Pediatrics.* 1987;80:750–751
4. Education of the Handicapped Act Amendments of 1986. *Federal Register.* October 1986
5. American Academy of Pediatrics (1989). Proceedings from a National Conference on Public Law 99-457: physician participation in the implementation of the law; November 19–21; Washington, DC.

# AMERICAN ACADEMY OF PEDIATRICS

# Physician's Role in Coordinating Care of Hospitalized Children

Committee on Hospital Care                    (RE9634)

**ABSTRACT.** This statement reminds physicians, hospitals, and other organizations (eg, review organizations or insurance companies) of existing guidelines that are important when children are hospitalized.

Today the most common reasons for hospitalization of children are acute illnesses or injuries and exacerbations of chronic illnesses or conditions. The length of hospital stay continues to decrease as more sophisticated care is delivered on an outpatient basis. Great emphasis is being placed on discharging children from the hospital as early as possible. Although hospital costs may be reduced as a result, the shortened stay may curtail a thorough evaluation. This may be detrimental to the child's welfare.

For all children needing hospital admission, whether in a community hospital, a rehabilitation hospital, or a children's hospital with all levels of care, an initial assessment must be made before or at the time of hospitalization. This evaluation enables children to be admitted to the inpatient unit that is best suited for their specific problems. At times the need for care may be met best by admission to a short-stay unit. If the inpatient unit best suited to the child's needs is not on the approved list of the child's insurance carrier, the physician needs to advocate for the best interest of the child and seek approval for admission to the appropriate unit.

A complete evaluation includes a history of present illness; general medical history; review of immunizations; developmental, educational, and emotional status; social and family history; and a physical examination including growth and developmental assessment.[1(pp121–122)] The effect of the child's condition on his or her family and the effect of the family on the child's condition need to be evaluated. This assessment may be done just before or concurrent with hospitalization.

It is especially important that the child's medical history is obtained from the primary care physician. Pediatric subspecialists or surgeons who hospitalize children with complex or multiple problems must communicate or consult with the child's primary pediatrician for overall coordination of care (including obtaining authorization if necessary). For children with chronic illnesses or past hospitalizations, hospital records must be available on admission for the health care team to review. Access to these

records prevents unnecessary duplication of prior interventions, allows physicians to update the status of past conditions that may not be obvious on this admission, and enables them to monitor the child's growth and developmental changes.

Before discharge, an assessment of the child's needs can be made, plans formulated, treatment provided, and necessary information supplied to the family members. Plans and treatments must be in accordance with the child's developmental, educational, and emotional level. Family members must be informed of the physician's recommended treatment plan because they are ultimately responsible for the informed decision about the care their child receives.

If plans for treatment are not completed during the hospitalization, appropriate outpatient management must be arranged. The child's social, developmental, and family status are particularly important because most children will receive part of their treatment on an outpatient basis. The physician is responsible for evaluating whether the outpatient treatment plan appears feasible for the child's family to undertake and modifying the plan if needed. At the time of discharge, a written summary and recommendations for outpatient care must be available to all personnel involved in the future care of the child. Referrals must be provided for all needed outpatient services, including a source of primary care if the child does not have a primary physician.[2,3] All referrals for outpatient services should be to physicians or organizations familiar with the special needs of children.

Occasionally the child's physician, when determining the need for inpatient care, may not be in agreement with decisions made by external organizations (eg, review organizations or insurance companies). Standards of medical care established by peer groups should be used as guidelines when controversy exists. In such situations, treatment and discharge decisions must be made with the best interests of the child as the primary motivation.[1(pp217–218)]

COMMITTEE ON HOSPITAL CARE, 1995 TO 1996
James E. Shira, MD, Chairperson
Jess Diamond, MD
Mary E. O'Connor, MD
John M. Packard, Jr, MD
Russell C. Raphaely, MD
Marleta Reynolds, MD
Henry A. Schaeffer, MD

LIAISON REPRESENTATIVES
C. Stamey English, MD
    American Academy of Family Physicians

PEDIATRICS (ISSN 0031 4005). Copyright © 1996 by the American Academy of Pediatrics.

Mary T. Perkins, RN, DNSC
Society of Pediatric Nurses
Mark A. Wallace
American Hospital Association
Jerriann M. Wilson
Association for the Care of Children's
Health
Paul S. Kramer
National Association of Children's
Hospitals and Related Institutions
Paul R. VanOstenberg, DDS, MS
Joint Commission on Accreditation of
Healthcare Organizations

AAP SECTION LIAISON
Theodore Striker, MD
Section on Anesthesiology

## REFERENCES

1. *1995 Comprehensive Accreditation Manual for Hospitals.* Oak Brook Terrace, IL: Joint Commission on Accreditation of Healthcare Organizations; 1994
2. American Academy of Pediatrics, Ad Hoc Task Force on Definition of the Medical Home. The medical home. *Pediatrics.* 1992;90:774
3. American Academy of Pediatrics. Pediatric primary health care. *AAP News.* 1993;November:7

# AMERICAN ACADEMY OF PEDIATRICS

## Provision of Related Services for Children With Chronic Disabilities

(RE9339)

Committee on Children With Disabilities

Since 1975 all children with disabilities specifically delineated by law have had available to them "a free, appropriate public education that includes special education and related services to meet their unique needs." This access has been made possible by the passage of Public Law 94-142,[1] The Education for All Handicapped Children Act of 1975. This law was amended in October 1990 with passage of Public Law 101-476, The Individuals With Disabilities Education Act (IDEA). Part B of Public Law 101-476 primarily details the identification and provision of services for children with disabilities. Unfortunately, the implementation of Part B of this law has been limited for many children by a number of significant and complex issues.

The term "related services" as currently defined in Part B of the IDEA includes the following:

... transportation and such developmental, corrective, and other supportive services (including speech pathology and audiology, psychological services, physical and occupational therapy, recreation and social work services, and medical and counseling services, including rehabilitation counseling, except that such medical services shall be for diagnostic and evaluation purposes only) as may be required to assist a child with a disability to benefit from special education.

Health care providers frequently view the related services listed above as medically necessary and/or helpful for children with disabilities without the proviso that these services must be necessary for special education. This difference in perspective and interpretation by pediatricians and parents often leads to misunderstandings, frustrations, conflicts, and problems in the development and implementation of related services within school programs for children with disabilities. To best serve children with disabilities and their families, pediatricians need to be familiar with these issues, their legal basis, and the special educational process and system.

Providing related services presents significant opportunities for the children served and challenges for the educational system. With an increasing number of children with chronic diseases and disabling conditions entering the school system and the increasing complexity of these conditions, many issues and problems have developed. The availability of services, designation of responsibility for their payment and provision, and conflicting legal imperatives as

well as other obstacles may ultimately prevent children from receiving potentially beneficial and needed services. Finally, the current trend of integration and inclusion of many children with a wide range of disabilities in "regular" classrooms and programs will make the provision of related services outside of traditional "special" educational settings a larger and more complex future issue.

The difficulties in implementation of Public Law 101-476 are as varied and complicated as the disabilities of the children involved. Among others, these problems include[2-4] (1) lack of clarity as to what circumstances should result in a child's exclusion from school for medical reasons; (2) uncertainty concerning responsibility for and/or administration of medical treatment in school; (3) inconsistencies in state and local guidelines and interpretations regarding who can and should prescribe the type and amount of physical, occupational, and speech therapies; (4) uncertainty about medical liability for therapies administered in school; (5) conflicting opinions concerning the propriety of some therapies being used for children; (6) concern about the rising cost of special education services and whether all treatment recommended in Individual Education Plans (IEPs) is warranted; and (7) the lack of provision of related services for children who may not require special education but who have chronic disabilities that impair their ability and readiness to attend and/or participate in school.

This statement primarily addresses the problem of children with chronic disabilities who may not require special education and the lack of provision of related services for them. For families and health care providers who believe that related services are desired and/or necessary, other legal justifications exist both within and beyond Public Law 101-476.

### ISSUES

While initially it seems clear within the above definition that related services are those necessary to aid a child with a disability to benefit from special education, there are a number of additional conflicting issues. These conflicts exist as a result of additional amendments to IDEA, as well as Section 504 of the Rehabilitation Act of 1973, and a variety of court rulings.

In 1986, Public Law 94-142 was amended through the enactment of Public Law 99-457 (and its subsequent reauthorization, as Public Law 102-119, which included Part H programs for infants and toddlers with disabilities). The purpose of Part H is to strengthen incentives for "statewide comprehensive

This statement has been approved by the Council on Child and Adolescent Health.

The recommendations in this policy statement do not indicate an exclusive course of treatment or serve as a standard of medical care. Variations, taking into account individual circumstances, may be appropriate.

PEDIATRICS (ISSN 0031 4005). Copyright © 1993 by the American Academy of Pediatrics.

coordinated multidisciplinary interagency program(s) of early intervention services for all infants and toddlers with disabilities and their families." In effect, implementation of Part H extends the availability of services to infants and toddlers with disabilities and their families from birth. Part H specifies the services to be those necessary to meet the developmental needs of each eligible child and the family needs related to enhancing the child's development in conformity with an Individualized Family Service Plan (IFSP). The IFSP is developed through evaluations assessing the following five domains: physical development; cognitive development; communication development; social or emotional development; and/or adaptive development. The philosophy behind providing these services is to maximize the developmental potential of these children and their families. This process recognizes the potential global benefits of these services, even if that child has deficits in a single domain (for example, physical development) and therefore may not require special educational or cognitive services.

While there are many similarities, significant inconsistencies exist between Part B and Part H in the requirements governing the provision of related services. Part H specifically includes interventions that under Part B are defined as related services without the restriction that the child receives special education (cognitive services). In fact, those services defined as related services in Part B are considered primary interventions in Part H. It makes little sense to consider services such as speech, physical, or occupational therapy important components of a program for a child younger than 3 years of age, but not necessarily important for a child older than 3 years of age unless the child's needs have changed. A change in the focus or location of the agency providing these services does not lessen the child's need for services. Children with chronic diseases and disabling conditions are best served by the acknowledgment of the consistency of their needs at all ages, rather than by the inconsistency of service delivery created by these statutes and regulations.

A further legal justification for the provision of related services without special class placement can be found in Section 504 of the Rehabilitation Act of 1973. This section prohibits discrimination on the basis of disability within federal and federally assisted programs. Regulations promulgated by the Department of Education have more broadly defined both the individuals covered by this act as well as the services that are to be provided. According to Section 504, all children should be provided with an appropriate education that "could consist of education in regular classes, education in regular classes with the use of supplementary services, or special educational and related services." Psychological testing and evaluation, counseling, physical and occupational therapy, medical services, speech pathology, audiology, and orientation mobility instruction are listed among the types of "developmental, corrective, and . . . support services" that may be provided to qualified individuals. Thus, Section 504 implies that children with special needs are entitled to appropriate modifications within their educational program to accommodate their special needs, regardless of whether their classroom placement is considered regular education or special education.

Court rulings have generally mandated that therapies recommended in the IEP be reimbursed by the educational system.[5] However, this has not precluded the application of Medicaid or other public funding to support medical service provisions for the disabled child. While private insurance carriers have generally declined to reimburse for therapies provided in the schools, in specific situations they can be responsible for payment of such services. The parents, however, have the right to decline to make claims against their insurance if it would create a realistic threat of financial loss by, for example, lowering the child's available lifetime medical benefits. Since the school systems have been bearing the responsibility for implementation of the IEP and funding most of the therapies, the educational authorities have increasingly been concerned with the responsibility for overseeing the delivery of medical care and other related services for disabled children attending public school. The assumption of these responsibilities has the potential to (1) increase conflicts with local physicians and other agencies responsible for health care delivery; (2) contribute to the disjointed nature of health care for children; and (3) result in unnecessary treatment at increased cost.[6]

The physician's role is currently defined as a related service and is interpreted to be diagnostic and consultative only. This interpretation becomes problematic in its failure to recognize the physician's role in the medical management, supervision, and program planning process for these children. The lack of physician input on treatment-related issues has posed the following important questions: (1) Does the health or the education system have the primary responsibility to oversee the delivery of health-related services in the school? (2) From what source should payment for such services be derived—educational funds, health-related entitlement programs, public health funding, or third-party insurers?

## CONCLUSION

Just as a multidisciplinary approach is mandated and necessary in the initial evaluation of children to determine their eligibility for services within the educational system, it is necessary to maintain a comprehensive, multidisciplinary approach in the provision of these services. The inequalities in the interpretation and provision of services between and within states, and even school districts, present a cogent reason for clear, equitable interpretation of Public Law 101-476. Providing related services for children who may not receive special educational services and allowing for greater medical involvement may require new models of interaction and collaboration between the medical and educational systems. However, the increasing number of children with complex medical needs now within the educational system and the more frequent inclusion of these children within regular programs is blurring the distinction between medical and educational services and regular and special educational services. There is an increasing amount of data to suggest subtle impairments in the school performance of children with chronic conditions who might otherwise appear to be intellectually unaffected.[7] The requirement of special educational services as the entree for other services implies that schools are to provide only cognitive educational services and that children do not learn from, need, or benefit from other school services and activities. This assumption is narrow and inconsistent with current thought and the provision of a free and appropriate education for children with disabilities because it does not adequately address the unique and complex total needs of these children. Providing these children with related services by utilizing a comprehensive approach to their chronic and disabling conditions will afford them the best opportunity to achieve their maximum potential.

## RECOMMENDATIONS

1. The focus for services should be on the child with a disability and his or her specific needs, not the relationship of these services to the child's educational placement. The specific class placement should not determine the provision of related services in school. Health care providers need to be aware of the issues and inconsistencies in Public Law 101-476, Parts B and H, and Section 504 of the Rehabilitation Act of 1973. Such an awareness will enable them to serve as effective providers, resources, and advocates for children with disabilities and their families. This should help ensure that children with disabilities who do not have significant cognitive or achievement impairments, but would benefit from related services, would more likely have their total educational needs met.

2. It is important that physicians, especially pediatricians, seek representation on the local advisory and interagency committees that oversee programs for placement of children with disabilities in schools. This would allow physicians to take a more active role in the development and implementation of the IEP process.

3. To be effective in overseeing the provision of services, including related services, physicians should be well informed concerning the needs of children with disabilities. Educational opportunities about these issues should be made readily available for interested physicians.

4. The supervision of medical care and health-related services for children with chronic and disabling conditions is the responsibility of physicians and the medical community, regardless of the location or source of payment for these services. When this oversight responsibility extends to services provided by the school system, clear and careful collaboration and coordination with the educational authorities is necessary. Issues such as the source of payment, liability, location(s) for treatment, and the specific staff performing the treatment(s) should be resolved with the responsible state and local agencies.

5. The Academy recommends that the potential for the physician's role in the care of children with disabilities within the schools be expanded by revising and clarifying the definition of medical services. The child, his or her family, and the school may benefit by medical consultation to determine and supervise specific medical, nursing, and therapy needs of the child within the educational setting. Medical services should not be limited to diagnosing the child's medically related disabling condition that results in the need for special education and related services. Medical services should be defined to encompass diagnosis, evaluation, consultation, and the medical supervision of those other services that are by statute, regulations, and/or professional traditions the responsibility of a licensed physician.

Committee on Children With Disabilities, 1993 to 1994
James Perrin, MD, Chair
Gerald Erenberg, MD
Ruth K. Kaminer, MD
Robert La Camera, MD
John A. Nackashi, MD
John R. Poncher, MD
Virginia Randall, MD
Renee C. Wachtel, MD
Philip R. Ziring, MD

Liaison Representatives
Connie Garner, RN, MSN, EdD, US Dept of Education Programs
Ross Hays, MD, American Academy of Physical Medicine and Rehabilitation
Joseph G. Hollowell, MD, Centers for Disease Control and Prevention, Center for Environmental Health and Injury Control
Merle McPherson, MD, Maternal and Child Health Bureau, Dept of Health and Human Services

Section Liaison
Harry L. Gewanter, MD, Section on Rheumatology

## REFERENCES

1. The Education for All Handicapped Children Act of 1975. 20 USC §1400 et seq
2. Bergdorf RL. *The Legal Rights of Handicapped Persons, Case Materials, Test.* Baltimore, MD: Paul H. Brookes Publishing Co; 1980
3. Wright GF. The pediatrician's role in Public Law 94-142. *Pediatr Rev.* 1982;4:191–197
4. Low MB. The Education for All Handicapped Children Act of 1975: a pediatrician's viewpoint. *Pediatrics.* 1978;62:271–274
5. *North v District of Columbia Board of Education.* 471 F suppl 136 (DC 1979). ELHR 1979;551:157
6. Palfrey JS, Singer JD, Raphael ES, Walker DK. Providing therapeutic services to children in special educational placements: an analysis of the related services provisions of Public Law 94-142 in five urban school districts. *Pediatrics.* 1990;85:518–525
7. Stoff E, Bacon MC, White PH. The effects of fatigue, distractibility, and absenteeism on school achievement in children with rheumatic diseases. *Arthritis Care Res.* 1989;2:49–53

## SUGGESTED READINGS

1. Horne RL. The education of children and youth with special needs: what do the laws say? *NICHCY News Digest* 1991;1:1
2. Kupper L, ed. Related services for school-aged children with disabilities. *NICHCY News Digest.* 1991;1:2

# AMERICAN ACADEMY OF PEDIATRICS

## Psychosocial Risks of Chronic Health Conditions in Childhood and Adolescence (RE9338)

Committee on Children With Disabilities and Committee on Psychosocial Aspects of Child and Family Health

Chronic health conditions affect many children and adolescents. These conditions are illnesses or impairments that are expected to last for an extended period of time and require medical attention and care that is above and beyond what would normally be expected for a child or adolescent of the same age, extensive hospitalization, or in-home health services.[1] These conditions include, among others, juvenile rheumatoid arthritis, asthma, cystic fibrosis, diabetes, spina bifida, hemophilia, seizure disorders, neuromuscular disease, acquired immunodeficiency syndrome, and congenital heart diseases. Although each specific condition may be relatively or extremely rare, when they are considered together, many children and adolescents are affected.

Health conditions may be characterized by their *duration* and their *severity*. Although these terms are often linked, they refer to different aspects of a health condition. A chronic condition is generally one that has lasted or is expected to last more than a defined period of time, usually 3 months or longer. Conditions vary widely in their onset, course, and duration.[2] Severity refers to the impact a condition has on a child's physical, intellectual, psychological, or social functioning.[3] This impact may occur as a result of persistent symptoms, required treatments, limitations of activity or mobility, or interference with school, recreation, work, and family activities.

Current estimates are that between 10 and 20 million American children and adolescents have some type of chronic health condition or impairment. Most of these conditions are relatively mild and interfere little with the children's ability to participate in usual childhood activities.[4] However, at least 10% of children with chronic conditions, ie, approximately 2% of those aged 0 to 21 years (1½ to 2 million children and adolescents nationwide), have a chronic condition severe enough to have an impact on their daily lives.

Recent medical and surgical advances have markedly decreased the mortality rates for children and adolescents with chronic conditions. While previously many of these individuals died in childhood or adolescence, current data suggest that at least 90%, even those with severe conditions, survive at least to young adulthood.[5] Given this change in survival, health care for these children and adolescents must be expanded to include more than management of their chronic condition and intercurrent acute illnesses. Pediatric care should also maximize children's functional abilities and sense of well-being, their health-related quality of life, and their development into healthy and productive adults.

## PSYCHOLOGICAL RISKS OF CHRONIC CONDITIONS

Over the past two decades, much research has examined the psychological functioning of children and adolescents with various specific health conditions.[6] Large, community-based studies[7,8] and national surveys[9] have assessed the risk of emotional, behavioral, and educational difficulties experienced by children and adolescents with a chronic health condition. Most of these studies have examined parents' ratings of behavioral and emotional status and have not identified specific psychological disturbances. These studies suggest that the majority of children and adolescents with chronic health conditions do not have identifiable mental health, behavioral, or educational difficulties. Children and their families are remarkably resilient in adapting to the additional stresses and challenges presented by a chronic health condition. Children, their siblings, and their parents often learn new coping strategies and show evidence of exceptional strength and mastery as a result. Nevertheless, these same studies show that children and adolescents with chronic conditions do have about twice the prevalence of psychological symptoms as compared to children without a chronic condition. Behavioral or emotional symptoms can be identified in approximately 10% of children overall and in about 20% of children with chronic health conditions.

It is not clear which specific characteristics of the child or adolescent, the family, and the health condition itself contribute most to resilience, to the stresses experienced, and to the risk of developing secondary emotional or behavioral difficulties. One might expect that the more severe the condition is, the greater the likelihood of psychological problems. Most studies show surprisingly little, if any, relationship between severity and problems with psychological adjustment.[6,10,11] The risk of psychological adjustment problems seems to reflect more the presence of a chronic condition than its severity.[12] In general, the increased risk of psychological problems affects children and adolescents with all kinds of chronic conditions without great variation from one to another. There are characteristics of some conditions that do seem to be associated with higher rates of emotional or behavioral problems. For example, children who have chronic conditions that affect the central nervous system, especially seizure disorders,[7,9] and children and adolescents who have an associated long-term physical disability may be at a higher risk for psychological problems than children with other chronic conditions.[8] Dependence on others for daily activities may also contribute to their risk of psychosocial dysfunction. Specific health conditions may cause specific coping issues for children and adolescents, such as driving with epilepsy, issues involving sexuality for those with cystic fibrosis, or the social stigma of inflammatory bowel disease. However, children and adolescents with *any* type of chronic condition will have unique psychological stresses in addition to those faced by all children.

If neither the severity nor the type of condition adequately explains the risk of psychological problems, what family and child characteristics might predict this risk? Children's intelligence and temperament appear to contribute to their ability to adapt to the extra stresses of the illness.[13,14] Parents' self-esteem, mental health, social support network, and beliefs about health care all have an impact on the success of children's adaptation,[6,9,13,15] as does the cohesiveness, flexibility, and effectiveness of shared communication within the family. Current research efforts will likely identify additional factors associated with increased risks for psychological problems and factors that foster children's resilience. This information will provide pediatricians with more guidance regarding the prevention and identification of psychological difficulties when working with families whose children have chronic health conditions.

## RECOMMENDATIONS FOR PEDIATRIC CARE

Primary care pediatricians have a central role in providing screening, preventive, and supportive services to children and adolescents with chronic health conditions and their families.

The usual pediatric model of assessing children's functioning in their family, in school, and with peers applies to those with a chronic health condition just as it does to all other children and adolescents. Pediatricians who take a comprehensive and family-based view of the broad clinical implications of childhood chronic conditions will recognize their critical role in diminishing the child's risk of psychological adjustment problems. Identifying children and families at risk for coping poorly with the stress of chronic health problems; assisting families to prevent psychological, social, and behavioral complications; and searching for early evidence of such problems should be part of regular pediatric care. Most of the stressful issues for families with children with chronic conditions can be anticipated and dealt with preventively through education and supportive counseling services provided appropriately by the pediatrician. It may be appropriate for some children and adolescents to be referred for mental health services.

Pediatricians should develop links with local schools and other agencies that provide support and services for children and families. Schools play a central role in the education and socialization of all children and often have resources that help with the prevention, identification, and management of psychosocial problems in their students, including those with health impairments.[16] Because increasing numbers of children with chronic conditions are in school from the age of 3 years, schools are a key resource in their long-term management. They frequently provide major assistance to families and to pediatricians in diminishing the psychosocial risks of chronic conditions.

Pediatricians can also help families by ensuring well-coordinated medical care and efficient and effective communication with the many professional providers of care involved with the family. They can help to ensure that families have access to local supportive networks for parents and for children. Also, pediatricians should provide appropriate information about the individual's illness and its management, recreational opportunities, and mechanisms to assist with the financial strain associated with chronic health conditions.[17]

The prevention of psychosocial complications of childhood chronic illness will be met best by a family- and community-centered approach in which the pediatrician assesses the skills and needs of the child and family, participates in planning and implementing comprehensive intervention programs, and supports families in the complex task of raising children and adolescents with chronic conditions.[17]

Liaison Representative
Mervyn Fox, MD, Canadian Paediatric Society

Consultant
George J. Cohen, MD, National Consortium for
Child Mental Health Services

## REFERENCES

1. Pless IB, Pinkerton P. *Chronic Childhood Disorder: Promoting Patterns of Adjustment*. London, England: Kimpton; 1975
2. Perrin EC, Newacheck PW, Pless IB, et al. Issues involved in the definition and classification of chronic health conditions. *Pediatrics*. 1993;91: 787–793
3. Stein RE, Gortmaker SL, Perrin EC, et al. Severity of illness: concepts and measurements. *Lancet*. 1987;2:1506–1509
4. Gortmaker SL, Sappenfield W. Chronic childhood disorders: prevalence and impact. *Pediatr Clin North Am*. 1984;31:3–18
5. Newacheck PW. Adolescents with special health needs: prevalence, severity, and access to health services. *Pediatrics*. 1989;84:872–881
6. MacLean WE, Perrin JM, Gortmaker S, Pierre CB. Psychological adjustment of children with asthma: effects of illness severity and recent stressful life events. *J Pediatr Psychol*. 1992;17:159–171
7. Pless IB, Roghmann KJ. Chronic illness and its consequences: observations based on three epidemiologic surveys. *J Pediatr*. 1971;79:351–359
8. Cadman D, Boyle M, Szatmari P, Offord DR. Chronic illness, disability, and mental and social well-being: findings of the Ontario Child Health Study. *Pediatrics*. 1987;79:805–813
9. Gortmaker SL, Walker DK, Weitzman M, Sobol AM. Chronic conditions, socioeconomic risks, and behavioral problems in children and adolescents. *Pediatrics*. 1990;85:267–276
10. McAnarney ER, Pless IB, Satterwhite B, et al. Psychological problems of children with chronic juvenile arthritis. *Pediatrics*. 1974;53:523–528
11. Perrin JM, Maclean WE, Perrin EC. Parental perceptions of health status and psychologic adjustment of children with asthma. *Pediatrics*. 1989; 83:26–30
12. Hobbs N, Perrin JM, Ireys HT. *Chronically Ill Children and Their Families*. San Francisco, CA: Jossey-Bass; 1985
13. Perrin EC, Ayoub CC, Willett JB. In the eyes of the beholder: family and maternal influences on perceptions of adjustment of children with chronic illness. *J Dev Behav Pediatr*. 1993;14:94–105
14. Varni JW, Rubenfeld LA, Talbot D, Setoguchi Y. Family functioning, temperament, and psychologic adaptation in children with congenital or acquired limb deficiencies. *Pediatrics*. 1989;84:323–330
15. Stein RE, Jessop DJ. Relationship between health status and psychological adjustment among children with chronic conditions. *Pediatrics*. 1984; 73:169–174
16. American Academy of Pediatrics, Committee on Children With Disabilities and Committee on School Health. Children with health impairments in schools. *Pediatrics*. 1990;86:636–638
17. Brewer EJ, McPherson M, Magrab PR, Hutchins VL. Family-centered, community-based coordinated care for children with special health care needs. *Pediatrics*. 1989;83:1055–1060

# AMERICAN ACADEMY OF PEDIATRICS

# The Role of the Pediatrician in Implementing the Americans With Disabilities Act: Subject Review

Committee on Children With Disabilities      (RE9623)

**ABSTRACT.** In this statement, the American Academy of Pediatrics reaffirms the importance of the Americans With Disabilities Act (ADA), which guarantees people with disabilities certain rights to enable them to participate more fully in their communities. Pediatricians need to know about the ADA provisions to be able to educate and counsel their patients and patients' families appropriately. The ADA mandates changes to our environment, including reasonable accommodation to the needs of individuals with disabilities, which has application to schools, hospitals, physician offices, community businesses, and recreational programs. Pediatricians should be a resource to their community by providing information about the ADA and the special needs of their patients, assisting with devising reasonable accommodation, and counseling adolescents about their expanded opportunities under the ADA.

Pediatricians need to be aware of the potential implications of the Americans With Disabilities Act (ADA). The ADA, passed in 1990, guarantees people with disabilities certain rights that help include them in all aspects of community activities. In fact, the broad definition of disabilities covered by this act results in a significant (and increasing) percentage of pediatric patients potentially being able to use its provisions to participate more fully in their communities. Pediatricians need to understand the relevant sections of the law to educate and counsel parents and adolescent patients and to connect them with appropriate resources.

## ADA DEFINITION OF DISABILITY

The definition of a person with a disability for purposes of this legislation is someone who has a "physical or mental impairment that substantially limits one or more of the major life activities of said individual."[1] The ADA also covers individuals who were disabled previously or treated as if they were, even if currently they are not. The regulations do not supply a list of impairments but specify that any physiologic disorder or condition affecting one or more body systems is included if it interferes with life activities. This definition includes limitation in the "manner or duration" of the performance of a life activity and thus includes many common chronic diseases in pediatric patients, such as "contagious and noncontagious diseases, and conditions such as orthopedic, visual, speech, and hearing impairments, cerebral palsy, epilepsy, muscular dystrophy, diabetes, heart disease, specific learning disabilities, and HIV disease."[2]

Studies of the US National Health Interview Survey[3] have indicated that the percentage of children younger than 17 years identified with activity-limiting chronic conditions doubled (from 1.8% to 3.8%) between 1960 and 1981,[4] and data from the early 1990s indicate that rates have increased to more than 5%. This increase reflects a variety of factors, including increased survival of low birth weight infants, children with spinal cord and head trauma, and children with congenital disorders (eg, congenital heart disease or cystic fibrosis) previously associated with high mortality rates. In addition, an expanded view of the impact of common disorders (such as learning disabilities) in limiting major life activities has broadened the spectrum of children and adolescents potentially considered disabled under the ADA.

## ADA PROVISIONS

The ADA seeks to change, over time, the way people with disabilities participate in their communities, both by prohibiting discrimination and by requiring "reasonable adjustments" of the environment. Although the greatest application of its provisions may be for adults with disabilities, children and especially adolescents with disabilities can benefit significantly from its protections. The ADA serves to empower and enable people with disabilities to overcome or circumvent barriers that are frequently artificial.

Title III of the ADA describes the various public facilities and accommodations that are included in its antidiscrimination prohibitions. In contrast to the provisions of section 504 of the Rehabilitation Act, which requires an individual with disabilities to be "qualified" for the particular activity, job, or service, the ADA requires reasonable accommodation unless: (1) there would be an undue burden to do so; (2) it would fundamentally alter the service provided; or (3) the individual poses a direct threat to the health or safety of others. This "presumption of qualification" suggests that the public world belongs to all people.[5] Although other specific components of the ADA relate to public transportation, public accommodations, and housing, this statement focuses on access to public programs and services, communications, and employment.

This subject review has been approved by the Council on Child and Adolescent Health.

The recommendations in this statement do not indicate an exclusive course of treatment or serve as a standard of medical care. Variations, taking into account individual circumstances, may be appropriate.

PEDIATRICS (ISSN 0031 4005). Copyright © 1996 by the American Academy of Pediatrics.

## ACCESS TO PROGRAMS AND SERVICES

The provisions of the ADA apply to pediatric patients in many ways. The law prohibits discrimination against an individual on the basis of disability and the exclusion from participation in, or denial of the benefits of, the services, programs, and activities of a local government, including all public school system programs and activities. Because integration of individuals with and without recognized disabilities is fundamental to the ADA, state and local governments must provide services in the most integrated settings appropriate for the needs of the individual child, allowing interaction with children without disabilities to the greatest extent possible. Although specialized programs for children with disabilities may be offered, an individual with a disability cannot be denied the opportunity to participate in programs that are designed for individuals without impairments. For example, a child with a disability has the right to swim at a school pool without participating in a separate swimming program for children with disabilities.[6] In this situation, the school may impose legitimate safety requirements based on the actual risks associated with the particular child's disability, not on general presumptions about individuals with that type of disability. Furthermore, the wishes or preferences of teachers or children cannot justify denying children with disabilities participation in programs or activities that use the school swimming pool or gym. School systems must provide wheelchair access for children with disabilities, although it is not required that every school be wheelchair accessible.

## COMMUNICATIONS

The telecommunications provisions of the ADA are particularly important for middle school children and adolescents with hearing impairments. At these ages, socialization skills frequently include telephone communication that connects them with peers without disabilities. Title IV of the ADA requires each state to have a telephone relay system that provides an interface between hearing and nonhearing and speech-impaired communicators, which increases the functional independence of impaired communicators and gives them a sense of belonging to their peer group.

## ACCESS TO OTHER SERVICES

One important provision of the ADA is the requirement that individuals with disabilities have access to programs and services generally available to other members of the public. Such provisions affect almost all community businesses, such as restaurants, banks, retail stores, and medical offices. Programs and services must make needed accommodations, except when doing so creates an undue financial burden. Generally, freight elevators, back doors, or carrying the individual would not be considered effective access, unless used as a last resort and comparable to the access of individuals without disabilities. Expenditures for accommodations do not need to be exorbitant. The law specifically states that costs need to be reasonable in the context of the resources of the business. Furthermore, the majority of the adjustments and accommodations are inexpensive, require little or no building renovations, and can be readily accomplished.

## EMPLOYMENT PROVISIONS

The ADA provides specific requirements regarding employment of people with disabilities. These requirements include physician offices and hospitals, among essentially all other employers, although the effective date of compliance varies according to the number of employees. These provisions benefit adolescents with disabilities by prohibiting discrimination when they seek part-time jobs during their school years and for career planning as they join the adult work force. Physician offices, health centers, and hospitals have expanded opportunities to hire employees with disabilities who can serve as role models for younger patients with disabilities using these services.

## CONCLUSION

The ADA guarantees civil rights to children and adolescents with disabilities and their families and mandates changes to our environment to enable the equal participation and reasonable accommodation of those with disabilities. Pediatricians can increase community sensitivity to the provisions of the ADA by being advocates for their patients with disabilities. Because children learn to become autonomous through interactions with the environment (both physical and psychological), modifications in the community may need to be made to encourage and support learning for those with disabilities to achieve functional independence.[7] Further information about the ADA is available in the reference list,[8,9] and from the ADA information centers in each region. Also, a resource packet is available from the American Academy of Pediatrics Department of Health Policy and State Advocacy.

COMMITTEE ON CHILDREN WITH DISABILITIES, 1994 TO 1995
James Perrin, MD, Chair
Gerald Erenberg, MD
Robert La Camera, MD
John A. Nackashi, MD
John R. Poncher, MD
Virginia Randall, MD
Elizabeth Ruppert, MD
Renee C. Wachtel, MD
Philip R. Ziring, MD

LIAISON REPRESENTATIVES
Polly Arango
    Family Voices
Debbie Gaebler, MD
    American Academy of Physical Medicine and Rehabilitation
Connie Garner, RN, MSN, EdD
    US Dept of Education Programs
Diane Garro
    Social Security Administration

Joseph G. Hollowell, MD
  Centers for Disease Control and Prevention
  Center for Environmental Health and Injury
  Control
John Mather, MD
  Social Security Administration
Merle McPherson, MD
  Maternal and Child Health Bureau
  Department of Health and Human Services
SECTION LIAISON
Harry L. Gewanter, MD
  Section on Rheumatology

## REFERENCES

1. The Americans With Disabilities Act of 1990, 42 USC §12102. Pub L No. 101-336
2. US Department of Justice. Nondiscrimination on the basis of disability by public accommodations and in commercial facilities. In: *Codes of Federal Regulations*. Washington, DC: Office of the Federal Register, National Archives and Records Administration; 1994;28:467–643
3. Newacheck PW, Budetti PP, Halfon N. Trends in activity limiting chronic conditions among children. *Am J Public Health*. 1986;76:178–184
4. Newacheck PW, Taylor WR. Childhood chronic illness: prevalence, severity, and impact. *Am J Public Health*. 1992;82:364–371
5. Parmet WE. Title III—public accommodations. In: Gostin LO, Beyer HA, eds. *Implementing the Americans With Disabilities Act. Rights and Responsibilities of All Americans*. Baltimore, MD: Brookes Publishing Co; 1993:123–136
6. Kilb L. Title II—Public services, subtitle A. In: Gostin LO, Beyer HA, eds. *Implementing the Americans With Disabilities Act. Rights and Responsibilities of All Americans*. Baltimore, MD: Brookes Publishing Co; 1993:87–108
7. Kalscheur JA. Benefits of the Americans With Disabilities Act of 1990 for children and adolescents with disabilities. *Am J Occup Ther*. 1992;46:419–426
8. Pope AM, Tarlov AR, Institute of Medicine. *Disability in America: Toward a National Agenda for Prevention*. Washington, DC: National Academy Press; 1991
9. West J, ed. The Americans With Disabilities Act: from policy to practice. *Milbank Q*. 1991;69(suppl 1-2):3–360

# AMERICAN ACADEMY OF PEDIATRICS

## The Role of the Pediatrician in Prescribing Therapy Services for Children With Motor Disabilities

Committee on Children With Disabilities          (RE9629)

**ABSTRACT.** Pediatricians are often called upon to prescribe physical and occupational therapy service for children with motor disabilities. This statement defines the context in which rehabilitation therapies should be prescribed, emphasizing the identification and enhancement of the child's function and abilities. The statement encourages the pediatrician to work with teams including the parents, child, teachers, therapists, and other physicians.

Pediatricians commonly are asked to evaluate children with motor disabilities and to write prescriptions for physical and occupational therapy. Although many states require a physician's prescription for such services, many physicians have limited formal education about these therapeutic interventions.[1]

The spectrum of motor impairments affecting function in children and adolescents includes acquired spinal injury, traumatic brain injury, muscular dystrophy, arthrogryposis, spina bifida, and cerebral palsy. Many children with these conditions will benefit from physical or occupational therapy.

Although physical and occupational therapy are often components of the treatment programs for children with disabilities, no current evidence indicates that these therapies directly improve the specific motor impairment of the child.[2–6] Rather, therapists, working with the family, child, and teacher, promote a positive functional adaptation to the disability in the context of the child's developmental progress. In the last decade, some treatment programs for children with cerebral palsy and other motor disabilities have been carefully evaluated using meta-analysis, functional measures, and single-subject design methods.[7–12] Clear documentation of efficacy has continued to be elusive. This problem may in part reflect difficult issues of methodology associated with the study of therapeutic efficacy in children because of their changing maturation and the need to identify and measure appropriate outcome criteria.[2–4] A meta-analysis of 31 studies of early intervention found higher performance scores for children receiving services compared with a control group, with greater effects on overall developmental quotients than on specific measures of motor function. In one important study, physical therapy alone was found to be less effective than the incorporation of developmentally appropriate play and learning skills for motor-impaired children younger than 3 years.[12]

Given the multiple needs of the child with a disability, one therapeutic discipline alone rarely minimizes the effects of the disability. Well-controlled scientific studies with well-defined functional outcome measurements are therefore necessary to clarify the efficacy of physical and occupational therapy interventions for specific pediatric conditions. Issues such as the frequency and intensity of therapy services, the relationship to assistive technology, and rehabilitative and medical versus developmental models of therapy all require further investigation.

The pediatrician needs to understand the role of physical and occupational therapists in the overall treatment of children with disabilities and the therapeutic modalities that may affect functioning and otherwise help these children.[13–16] Physical therapists focus on gross motor skills, including sitting; sitting to standing in preparation for transfers; walking with or without assistive devices and braces; wheelchair propulsion; transfers out of the wheelchair (to a desk, toilet, or bath); negotiation of ramps, curbs, and elevators; and problem-solving skills for accessibility of public buildings. Physical therapists often have responsibilities for ordering equipment and assistive devices.[17–19] Occupational therapists focus on fine motor and visual motor skills that improve the integrated activities of daily living, such as dressing, grooming, toileting, eating, bathing, and writing.[20,21] Occupational therapy services may also include training in school readiness skills and the identification of techniques to help children compensate for specific deficits. Occupational therapists also provide expert consultation on certain technologies, such as environmental control units, augmentative communication systems, and adaptive toys.[20] If the child has motor problems severe enough to interfere with self-care or communication, the therapist may recommend a program to help the child compensate for the disability or adapt to it. Despite anecdotal reports of beneficial results in selected cases, however, neurophysiologic retraining programs that purport to alter the underlying neurologic disorder have little effect on functional skills and are inappropriate for children with motor disabilities.[5,6,22] Participation in sports can increase their endurance, self-esteem, and strength in a peer setting.[23]

This statement has been approved by the Council on Child and Adolescent Health.

The recommendations in this statement do not indicate an exclusive course of treatment or serve as a standard of medical care. Variations, taking into account individual circumstances, may be appropriate.

PEDIATRICS (ISSN 0031 4005). Copyright © 1996 by the American Academy of Pediatrics.

The pediatrician's primary responsibility in writing a prescription for therapy is to provide an accurate diagnosis. Although often the cause of the disability is not apparent, the physician must provide an accurate description of the medical condition and whether the child has a transient, static, or progressive impairment. In addition to the primary neuromotor disorder, all potential associated problems, such as learning disabilities, mental retardation, sensory impairment, speech disorders, emotional difficulties, and seizure disorders, must be identified, and treatment must be recommended. Children with medical conditions that may be adversely affected by movement or other specific activities should have those conditions identified as precautions. Occupational and physical therapists cannot make determinations on drug treatment and the children's medical risks during therapy. For example, weight-lifting activity during therapy may be contraindicated in some children with motor disabilities receiving long-term prednisone therapy because of the increased risk of fracture(s). Medical precautions may reflect cardiovascular parameters, seizure precautions, or range-of-motion precautions.

The prescription for therapy should designate its goals. Plans for physical and occupational therapy do not depend solely on the diagnosis or age of the patient. They are most appropriate when developed to address specific functional goals in individual patients. The pediatrician should work with the family, child, therapist, school personnel, developmental diagnostic team, and other physicians to establish realistic functional goals.[24,25] The pediatrician can help families develop expectations of the goals of treatment and help them understand that treatment mainly assists in their adaptation to a condition rather than changing the underlying neuromuscular problem. Pediatricians should be able to contact and use expert consultation as in any other area of medicine. Helpful resources include local and regional diagnostic teams, early intervention and developmental evaluation programs, developmental pediatricians, pediatric physiatrists, and pediatric neurologists.

Therapy prescriptions should contain the child's diagnosis, precautions, type of therapy, frequency of therapy, anticipated goals, and duration of therapy. Two examples of prescriptions include:

1. Diagnosis: cerebral palsy, spastic quadriplegia, severe dysphagia
   Precautions: risk of aspiration with seizure
   Type and frequency of therapy: speech therapy 2x/week × 6 mos
   Improve oral motor stimulation and provide a desensitization home program
   Goal: improve oral phase of swallowing to increase oral intake.
2. Diagnosis: complete C-7 quadriplegia
   Precautions: stable spine
   Type and frequency of therapy: physical therapy 2x/week × 6 mos
   Increased range of motion, increased strength in available muscles, increased trunk control

Goal: transfers without sliding board independently, between level surfaces, and propels wheelchair in household.

Successful programs require regular communication among the therapists, educators, and prescribing physicians, with periodic reevaluation to assess the achievement of identified goals, to direct therapy toward new objectives, and to determine when therapy is no longer warranted.[26] Therapies that are individually tailored to meet the child's functional needs should be integrated with the educational and medical treatment plans with consideration of the needs of parents and siblings.

### RECOMMENDATIONS

1. Pediatricians should be aware of all professionals and therapeutic modalities that have an impact on children with disabilities.
2. Pediatricians should be informed of and participate in setting functional goals for therapy.
3. Pediatricians should be involved with the ongoing process of evaluating therapy programs for children with disabilities.
4. Pediatricians should be aware of and use community resources, such as pediatric physiatry (rehabilitation medicine), local or regional diagnostic teams, and developmental pediatrics, to obtain expert consultation on therapeutic programs.

COMMITTEE ON CHILDREN WITH DISABILITIES, 1995 TO 1996
James Perrin, MD, Chair
Gerald Erenberg, MD
Robert La Camera, MD
John A. Nackashi, MD
John R. Poncher, MD
Virginia Randall, MD
Renee C. Wachtel, MD
W. Daniel Williamson, MD
Philip R. Ziring, MD

LIAISON REPRESENTATIVES
Polly Arango
    Family Voices
Deborah J. Gaebler-Spira, MD
    American Academy of Physical Medicine and Rehabilitation
Connie Garner, RN, MSN, EdD
    US Dept of Education Programs
Diana Garro
    Social Security Administration
Joseph G. Hollowell, MD
    Centers for Disease Control and Prevention
    Center for Environmental Health and Injury Control
John H. Mather, MD
    Social Security Administration
Merle McPherson, MD
    Maternal and Child Health Bureau
    Department of Health and Human Services

SECTION LIAISON
Harry Gewanter, MD
    Section on Rheumatology

### REFERENCES

1. Campbell SK, Anderson J, Gardner G. Physicians' beliefs in the efficacy of physical therapy in the management of cerebral palsy. *Pediatr Phys Ther.* 1990;2:169–173

2. Tirosh E, Rabino S. Physiotherapy for children with cerebral palsy: evidence for its efficacy. *Am J Dis Child.* 1989;143:522–525

3. Ottenbacher KJ. Efficacy of physical therapy: rate of motor development in children with cerebral palsy. *Pediatr Phys Ther.* 1990;2:131–134

4. Simeonsson RJ, Cooper DH, Scheiner AP. A review and analysis of the effectiveness of early intervention programs. *Pediatrics.* 1982;69:635–641

5. The Doman-Delacato treatment of neurologically handicapped children. *Pediatrics.* 1982;70:810–812

6. Carte E, Morrison D, Sublett J, Vemura A, Setrakian W. Sensory integration therapy: a trial of a specific neurodevelopmental therapy for the remediation of learning disabilities. *J Dev Behav Pediatr.* 1984;5:189–184

7. Harris SR. Efficacy of early intervention in pediatric rehabilitation: a decade of evaluation and review. *Phys Med Rehab Clin North Am.* 1991;2:725–742

8. Harris SR. Effects of neurodevelopmental therapy on motor performance of infants with Down's syndrome. *Dev Med Child Neurol.* 1981;23:477–483

9. Olney SJ. Efficacy of physical therapy in improving mechanical and metabolic efficiency of movement in cerebral palsy. *Pediatr Phys Ther.* 1990;2:145–154

10. Ottenbacher KJ, Biocca Z, DeCremer G, et al. Quantitative analysis of the effectiveness of physical therapy: emphasis on the neurodevelopmental treatment approach. *Phys Ther.* 1986;66:1095–1101

11. Shonkoff JP, Hauser-Cram P. Early intervention for disabled infants and their families: a quantitative analysis. *Pediatrics.* 1987;80:650–658

12. Palmer FB, Shapiro BK, Wachtel RC, et al. The effects of physical therapy on cerebral palsy: a controlled trial in infants with spastic diplegia. *N Engl J Med.* 1988;318:803–808

13. Consensus statements. *Pediatr Phys Ther.* 1990;2:175–176

14. Ottenbacher KJ, Peterson P. The efficacy of early intervention programs for children with organic impairment: a quantitative review. *Eval Program Plan.* 1985;8:135–146

15. Harris SR. Early intervention: does developmental therapy make a difference? *Topics Early Child Special Educ.* 1988;4:20–32

16. Piper MC. Efficacy of physical therapy: rate of motor development in children with cerebral palsy. *Pediatr Phys Ther.* 1990;2:126–130

17. Butler C. Effects of powered mobility on self-initiated behaviors of very young children with locomotor disability. *Dev Med Child Neurol.* 1986;28:325–332

18. Levangie P, Guihan MF, Meyer P, Stuhr K. Effect of altering handled position of a rolling walker on gait in children with cerebral palsy. *Phys Ther.* 1989;69:130–134

19. Taylor SJ. Evaluating the client with physical disabilities for wheelchair seating. *Am J Occup Ther.* 1987;41:711–716

20. Kibele A. Occupational therapy's role in improving the quality of life for persons with cerebral palsy. *Am J Occup Ther.* 1989;43:371–377

21. McCuaig M, Frank G. The able self: adaptive patterns and choices in independent living for a person with cerebral palsy. *Am J Occup Ther.* 1991;45:224–234

22. Ottenbacher K. Sensory integration therapy affect or effect? *Am J Occup Ther.* 1982;36:571–578

23. Johnstone K, Perrin J. Sports for the handicapped child. *Phys Med Rehab.* 1991;5:331–350

24. American Academy of Pediatrics, Committee on Children With Disabilities. The pediatrician's role in the development and implementation of an individual education plan. *Pediatrics.* 1987;80:750–751

25. American Academy of Pediatrics, Committee on Children With Disabilities. Pediatrician's role in the development of an individual education plan (IEP) and/or an individual family service plan (IFSP). *Pediatrics.* 1992;89:340–342

26. Levine M, Kliebhan L. Communication between physician and physical and occupational therapists: a neurodevelopmentally based prescription. *Pediatrics.* 1981;68:208–214

# AMERICAN ACADEMY OF PEDIATRICS

## The Role of the Primary Care Pediatrician in the Management of High-risk Newborn Infants (RE9636)

Committee on Practice and Ambulatory Medicine and Committee on Fetus and Newborn

**ABSTRACT.** Quality care for high-risk newborns can best be provided by coordinating the efforts of the primary care pediatrician and the neonatologist. This ideally occurs in the newborn period, during the critical care and convalescing periods, and through the time of discharge. This statement offers guidelines for the primary care pediatrician involved in providing neonatal care, and discusses his/her individual and shared responsibilities, roles, and relationships with the neonatologist and the neonatal intensive care unit.

Significant improvements in the successful treatment of high-risk newborns and critically ill neonates have been realized. These improvements have resulted from the rapid development of technology applied to the care of high-risk newborns and the regionalization of centers for the care of the critically ill newborn. These changes necessitate the primary care pediatrician having a better understanding of neonatal problems and the ability to coordinate patient care with the neonatologist. To prevent changes in the financing and delivery of health care services from jeopardizing the provision of vital high-risk newborn services, primary care pediatricians and neonatologists must develop an understanding of their individual and shared responsibilities. In this joint statement, the Committee on Practice and Ambulatory Medicine and the Committee on Fetus and Newborn of the American Academy of Pediatrics (AAP) address these concerns and offer guidelines for the primary care pediatrician involved in providing neonatal care.

Tertiary level centers should be staffed by full-time neonatalogists, while secondary level centers may be staffed by part-time neonatologists. The practice of neonatologists at these centers is usually based on referrals. It is the primary care pediatrician who makes the referrals to the neonatologist and who will assume responsibility for the case once critical care is no longer needed. Although the primary care pediatrician usually does not assume principal ongoing responsibility for the infant needing critical care, he or she should demonstrate expertise in several aspects of care of the seriously ill neonate.

## GUIDELINE I

In order to make timely decisions, the primary care pediatrician should be knowledgeable regarding problems that may occur in the perinatal period and should be able to accomplish the following:

1. Provide immediate and appropriate resuscitation and stabilization of the newborn infant. A critically ill neonate requires an organized plan of action and immediate availability of personnel and equipment as described in the *Textbook of Neonatal Resuscitation*,[1] published by the AAP and the American Heart Association.
2. Identify high-risk infants and conditions that may require specialized care. Examples include the following:

   - Cardiac disorders that require special diagnostic procedures or surgery
   - Gestational age less than 32 weeks or birth weight less than 1500 g
   - Suspected group B streptococcus infection, sepsis/meningitis, and other serious congenital infections
   - Infants not showing full recovery 6 hours after asphyxia
   - Congenital malformations requiring special diagnostic procedures or surgical care
   - Neonatal seizures
   - Conditions requiring exchange transfusions
   - Persistent or increasing respiratory distress beyond 1 hour of age
   - Infants failing to progress as expected in the neonatal period for any reason

   These examples are for use as guidelines only; consideration must be given to individual patient needs and institutional capabilities in implementation of the guidelines.

3. Determine which care option is suitable for a given case:

   - Newborn remaining in the care of the primary care pediatrician within a specialty or regular newborn nursery
   - Transfer of newborn to an intensive care setting
   - Consultation with a neonatologist to determine care options for the newborn
   - Transfer of the care of the newborn to a neonatologist.

## GUIDELINE II

The primary care pediatrician acts as an important communication link between the family and the personnel of the center providing critical care, whether or not they are both located in the same institution. In addition to providing support to the newborn's family, the primary care pediatrician should do the following:

1. The pediatrician should participate in the initial explanations of the medical problem(s) to the parents.
2. The pediatrician should facilitate the initial bonding process between the family and the newborn by arranging visitation time when possible and discussing the newborn's care with the parents.
3. The pediatrician should promote breastfeeding as the best nourishment for the ill or premature infant, and explore any reasons for choosing formula, in the event that this decision was based on misconception.
4. The pediatrician will sometimes serve as the major source of continuing information to parents, especially if the parents and the infant are separated by long distances. There may be instances in which it is desirable for the critical care personnel to communicate to the family primarily through the pediatrician.
5. The pediatrician should participate with the critical care personnel in discussions with the parents when a complicated course or poor outcome is expected.
6. The pediatrician should participate, when appropriate, in counseling the family with the neonatologist in the event the infant dies. When indicated, the pediatrician should arrange for genetic counseling.
7. The pediatrician should develop an awareness of the social, economic, or other factors that may have contributed to the high-risk state and communicate these to critical care personnel. These factors often continue into the period after treatment in the nursery; when appropriate, they should be taken into account in follow-up care.

There will be occasions where the primary care pediatrician will not previously know the family of the newborn or follow the infant after discharge. In such cases, it may be more appropriate to allow the neonatologist to assume some or all of the responsibilities as listed above, and allow the neonatologist to transition care to the family's chosen pediatrician toward the end of the hospitalization.

## GUIDELINE III

The primary care pediatrician should have the expertise to assume responsibility for the acute, though less critical, care of the infant. The convalescing newborn should be returned to the care of the primary care pediatrician, either when transferred back to the referring hospital or at the time of discharge home. The neonatologist and critical care personnel should communicate with the primary care physician to de-termine the appropriate timing of the return of the infant.

## GUIDELINE IV

The primary care pediatrician should understand the need for proper continuity of care and be capable of providing it through the following measures:

1. Identifying the problems created by the high-risk birth and postnatal disease. These may involve poor growth, pulmonary problems, developmental delays, hearing and vision deficits, risk of child abuse or neglect, behavior disturbances, and learning disabilities, as well as problems relating to initial heightened risk (eg, congenital anomalies). Other problems that may develop include those of family dynamics (eg, divorce) secondary to the stressful situation.
2. Ensuring access to hearing screening and retinal examinations for infants in accordance with AAP guidelines.[2,3]
3. Acting as a medical case manager for newborns who have multiple medical and/or developmental problems as a result of high-risk birth or postnatal disease or, if necessary, assist the family in linking with an appropriate case manager. The primary care pediatrician should be aware and be capable of utilizing community services for both the newborn and the family as the needs arise.
4. Providing feedback to the neonatologist regarding the developmental and medical outcomes of the child.
5. Using, as part of the program of longitudinal care, a systematic schema for the developmental and behavioral assessment of these infants through at least 7 to 10 years of age, as defined in the Academy's *Guidelines for Health Supervision II*.[4]
6. Sharing, when indicated, the responsibility of providing continuity of care with the tertiary or secondary care center. The center will often provide some of the developmental and psychologic evaluations and, perhaps, treatment programs that may not be otherwise available. Accurate and timely records of such services should be made available to the primary care pediatrician.
7. Becoming aware of and capable of dealing with the issues surrounding the "vulnerable child."

## GUIDELINE V

The primary care pediatrician should share responsibility with the neonatologist for the development and delivery of effective services in the hospital and community for newborns at risk through the following means:

1. Sharing, when appropriate, the responsibility for nursing and laboratory services as well as providing the appropriate equipment and facilities for emergency or continuing care of the infant at risk.
2. Participating in health care planning, collaborating with local obstetricians regarding standards of perinatal care, and participating in regular perinatal review conferences in each hospital. These conferences should include review of community

perinatal morbidity and mortality statistics, intensive care outcome data, and identification of areas of unmet need.

3. Participating on committees to develop effective community programs of staff training, infant transport, and public information.

4. Sharing with the neonatologist the responsibility for the education of other physicians and nonphysician health care providers regarding provision of quality health care to high-risk newborns.

The American Academy of Pediatrics therefore recommends that both the resident training and continuing education of the pediatrician continue to include the knowledge and the skills needed to provide appropriate primary and secondary level care for all newborns.

COMMITTEE ON PRACTICE AND AMBULATORY
MEDICINE, 1995 TO 1996
Peter D. Rappo, MD, Chair
Edward O. Cox, MD
John L. Green, MD
James W. Herbert, MD
E. Susan Hodgson, MD
James Lustig, MD
Thomas C. Olsen, MD
Jack T. Swanson, MD

SECTION LIAISONS
A. D. Jacobson, MD
  Section on Administration and Practice
  Management
Robert Sayers, MD
  Section on Uniformed Services
Julia Richerson Atkins, MD
  Resident Section

LIAISON REPRESENTATIVES
Todd Davis, MD
  Ambulatory Pediatric Association
Michael O'Neil, MD
  Canadian Paediatric Society

COMMITTEE ON FETUS AND NEWBORN, 1995 TO 1996
William Oh, MD, Chair
Lillian R. Blackmon, MD
Marilyn Escobedo, MD
Avroy A. Fanaroff, MD
Barry V. Kirkpatrick, MD
Irwin J. Light, MD
Hugh M. MacDonald, MD
Lu-Ann Papile, MD
Craig T. Shoemaker, MD

LIAISON REPRESENTATIVES
Michael F. Greene, Jr, MD
  American College of Obstetrics and Gynecologists
Patricia Johnson, RN, MS, NNP
  American Nurses Association, Association of
  Women's Health, Obstetric and Neonatal Nurses,
  National Association of Neonatal Nurses
Douglas D. McMillan, MD
  Canadian Paediatric Society
Diane Rowley, MD, MPH
  Centers for Disease Control and Prevention
Linda L. Wright, MD
  National Institutes of Health

AAP SECTION LIAISON
Jacob C. Langer, MD
  Surgical Section

## REFERENCES

1. American Academy of Pediatrics and American Heart Association. *Textbook of Neonatal Resuscitation.* Elk Grove Village, IL: American Academy of Pediatrics; 1995

2. American Academy of Pediatrics and American College of Obstetricians and Gynecologists. *Guidelines for Perinatal Care* (3rd ed). Washington, DC: American College of Obstetricians and Gynecologists; and Elk Grove Village, IL: American Academy of Pediatrics; 1992

3. American Academy of Pediatrics Joint Committee on Infant Hearing. 1994 Position statement. *Pediatrics.* 1995;95:152–155

4. American Academy of Pediatrics, Committee on Psychosocial Aspects of Child and Family Health. *Guidelines for Health Supervision II* (2nd ed). Elk Grove Village, IL: American Academy of Pediatrics; 1988

# AMERICAN ACADEMY OF PEDIATRICS

# Safe Transportation of Premature and Low Birth Weight Infants

Committee on Injury and Poison Prevention and Committee on Fetus and Newborn

(RE9617)

**ABSTRACT.** Special considerations are essential to ensure the safe transportation of premature and low birth weight infants. Both physical and physiologic issues must be considered in the proper positioning of these infants. This statement discusses current recommendations based on the latest research and provides guidelines for physicians who counsel parents of very small infants on the choice of the best car safety seats for their infants.

Improved survival rates and earlier discharge of premature infants have increased the number of infants weighing less than 2500 g who are being transported in private vehicles. To ensure that these infants are transported safely, specific guidelines regarding the proper selection and use of car safety seats and other occupant restraint devices for this population are warranted.

Currently, Federal Motor Vehicle Safety Standard 213, which established design and dynamic performance requirements for child restraint systems, applies to children weighing up to 50 lb but has no minimum weight limit established in the standard. Most safety restraints on the market are designed for infants weighing more than 7 lb (3.1 kg),[1,2] and only recently have studies been done that allow some prediction of the protective capabilities of restraint devices for infants weighing less than 7 lb. Research has indicated that some infants, particularly premature and low birth weight infants, may be subject to oxygen desaturation when placed in a semiupright position in car safety seats.[3–5] Both growth and neurologic maturation may influence the potential risk of respiratory compromise in seating devices. Further investigation is necessary to define precisely the population at risk and the situations in which risk occurs.

Several specific recommendations can be made regarding transportation of infants at possible risk of respiratory problems:

1. Current information suggests that each preterm infant born at less than 37 weeks' gestation should have a period of observation in a car safety seat before hospital discharge to monitor for possible apnea, bradycardia, or oxygen desaturation. An appropriate hospital staff person should conduct the observation. Hospitals should develop policies to include this evaluation in their discharge planning

process.[5] An Academy-endorsed video, "Special Delivery: Safe Transportation of Premature and Small Infants," contains additional information on this topic.[6]

2. Families should minimize travel for infants at risk of respiratory compromise.

3. Infants with documented desaturation, apnea, or bradycardia in a semiupright position should travel in a supine or prone position in an alternative safety device. The use of other upright equipment, including infant swings, infant seats, and infant carriers, should be avoided.

Alternative child restraint devices are available for infants who must travel in a prone, supine, or semiupright position. Specific information regarding currently available restraint systems can be obtained from the American Academy of Pediatrics brochure, "Family Shopping Guide to Car Seats."[7]

If a semiupright position can be maintained safely by the infant, a conventional car safety seat that allows for proper positioning of the low birth weight infant should be selected. Better observation of the infant is possible when the child is in a rear-facing car safety seat adjacent to an adult rather than in a car bed. (See guideline 7 in this statement for information on passenger-side front air bags.)

4. Infants for whom home cardiac and apnea monitors are prescribed should use this monitoring equipment during travel and have portable, self-contained power available for twice the duration of the expected transport time.

5. Because commercially available securement systems for all portable medical equipment such as monitors and oxygen tanks are limited and not designed for use in motor vehicles, such equipment should be wedged on the floor or under the vehicle seat to prevent it from becoming a dangerous projectile in the event of a crash or sudden stop.

Proper positioning of small infants in car safety seats is important to minimize the risk of respiratory compromise while providing protection in the event of a crash or sudden stop. Specific guidelines for selecting car safety seats and positioning small infants in them include the following:

1. Infant-only car safety seats with three-point harness systems or convertible car safety seats with five-point harness systems provide optimum comfort, fit, and positioning for the premature or small infant. A small infant should not be placed in a car safety seat with a shield, abdominal pad, or arm rest that could directly contact an infant's face and neck during an impact. Similarly, car safety seats designed

for use only by children who weigh more than 20 lb should not be used for small infants.

2. Car safety seats with a distance of less than 5½ in from the crotch strap to the seat back should be selected to reduce the potential of slumping forward of the low birth weight infant (Fig 1). A small rolled diaper or blanket between the crotch strap and the infant may be added to reduce slouching (Fig 2).

3. Car safety seats with a distance of less than 10 in from the lower harness strap to the seat bottom should be selected to reduce the potential of harness straps crossing the infant's ears (Fig 1).

4. The infant should be properly positioned in the car safety seat, with buttocks and back flat against the back of the car safety seat. Blanket rolls may be placed on both sides of the infant to provide lateral support for the head and neck (Fig 2).

5. In rear-facing car safety seats for infants, shoulder straps must be in the lowest slots until the infant's shoulders are above the slots; the harness must be snug; and the car safety seat's retainer clip should be positioned at the midpoint of the infant's chest, not on the abdomen or in the neck area (Fig 2).

6. If the vehicle seat slopes so that the infant's head flops forward, the car safety seat should be reclined halfway back, at a 45° tilt. Until engineering modifications can be implemented to prevent this problem, a firm roll of cloth or newspaper can be wedged under the car safety seat below the infant's feet to achieve this angle (Fig 3).

7. A rear-facing car safety seat must not be placed in the front passenger seat of any vehicle equipped with a passenger-side front air bag because of risk of death or serious injury from the impact of the air bag

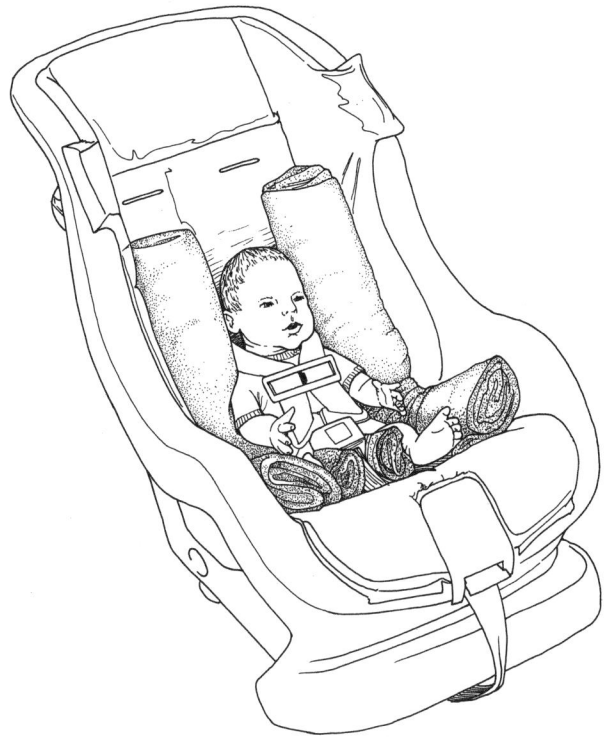

**Fig 2.** Car safety seat with retainer clip positioned on the infant's chest.

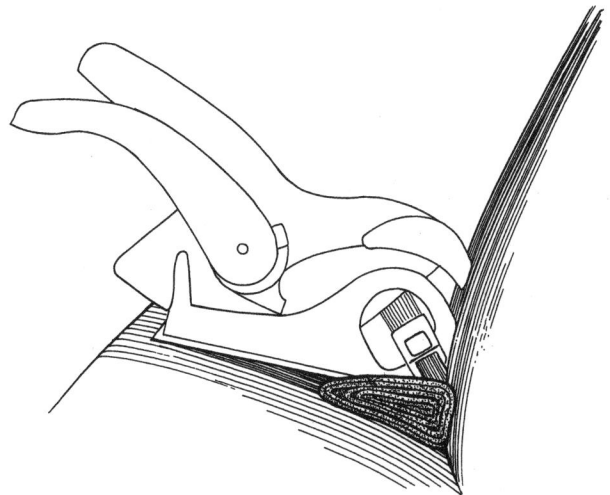

**Fig 3.** Seat with wedge to recline seat halfway back at a 45° tilt.

against the safety seat. All infants weighing less than 20 lb and younger than 1 year of age must ride rear facing when secured in standard car safety seats. Infants who weigh 20 lb before 1 year of age should ride rear facing in convertible seats or infant seats approved for higher weights until 1 year of age.[8] The rear seat is the safest position in which a child can ride in a vehicle, and whenever possible, parents should arrange for an adult to be seated in the rear seat adjacent to the infant to observe the child closely.

8. An infant should never be left unattended in a car safety seat.

The recommendations provided in this statement are proposed for premature and low birth weight

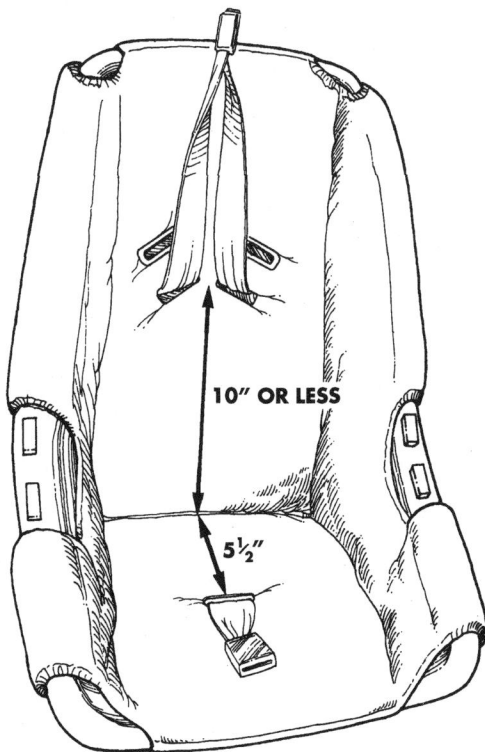

**Fig 1.** Car seat with a distance of 5½ in or less from the crotch strap to the seat back and 10 in or less from the lower harness strap to the seat bottom.

infants. The safe transportation of children with respiratory compromise due to neuromuscular and orthopedic problems is addressed in the policy statement, "Safe Transportation of Children With Special Needs."[9] Specific additional technical information on this topic also can be found in the Academy's speaker's and resource kit, "Child Restraint Systems: Getting It Right."[10]

COMMITTEE ON INJURY AND POISON PREVENTION, 1995 TO 1996
Murray L. Katcher, MD, PhD, Chair
Marilyn J. Bull, MD
S. Donald Palmer, MD
George C. Rodgers, Jr, MD, PhD
Barbara L. Smith, MD
Howard R. Spivak, MD
Susan B. Tully, MD

LIAISON REPRESENTATIVES
Phyllis Agran, MD, MPH
    Ambulatory Pediatric Association
Stephanie Bryn, MPH
    Maternal and Child Health Bureau
Dayle L. Maples, MD
    Pediatric Orthopaedic Society of North America
Cheryl Neverman
    US Dept of Transportation
Peter Scheidt, MD, MPH
    National Institute of Child Health and Human Development
Richard A. Schieber, MD, MPH
    Centers for Disease Control and Prevention
Milton Tenenbein, MD
    Canadian Paediatric Society
Deborah Tinsworth
    US Consumer Product Safety Commission

SECTION LIAISON
James Griffith, MD
    Section on Injury and Poison Prevention

COMMITTEE ON FETUS AND NEWBORN, 1995 TO 1996
William Oh, MD, Chair
Lillian R. Blackmon, MD
Marilyn Escobedo, MD
Avroy A. Fanaroff, MD
Barry V. Kirkpatrick, MD
Irwin J. Light, MD

Hugh M. MacDonald, MD
LuAnn Papile, MD
Craig T. Shoemaker, MD

LIAISON REPRESENTATIVES
Garris Keels Conner, RN, DSN
    American Nurses Association Association of Women's Health, Obstetric, and Neonatal Nurses National Association of Neonatal Nurses
James N. Martin, Jr, MD
    American College of Obstetricians and Gynecologists
Douglas D. McMillan, MD
    Canadian Paediatric Society
Diane Rowley, MD, MPH
    Centers for Disease Control and Prevention
Linda L. Wright, MD
    National Institute of Child Health and Human Development

AAP SECTION LIAISON
Jacob C. Langer, MD
    Section on Surgery

## REFERENCES

1. Bull MJ, Stroup KB. Premature infants in car seats. *Pediatrics*. 1985;75: 336–339
2. Bull MJ, Weber K, Stroup KB. Automotive restraint systems for premature infants. *J Pediatr*. 1988;112:385–388
3. Willett LD, Leuschen MP, Nelson LS, Nelson RM. Risk of hypoventilation in premature infants in car seats. *J Pediatr*. 1986;109:245–248
4. Willett LD, Leuschen MP, Nelson LS, Nelson RM. Ventilatory changes in convalescent infants positioned in car seats. *J Pediatr*. 1989;115: 451–455
5. Bass JL, Mehta KA, Camara J. Monitoring premature infants in car seats: implementing the American Academy of Pediatrics policy in a community hospital. *Pediatrics*. 1993;91:1137–1141
6. Automotive Safety for Children Program. *Special Delivery: Safe Transportation of Premature and Small Infants*. Indianapolis, IN: Automotive Safety for Children Program, Riley Hospital for Children; 1991. Videotape and booklet
7. American Academy of Pediatrics. *Family Shopping Guide to Car Seats: 1996*. Elk Grove Village, IL: American Academy of Pediatrics; 1996. Brochure
8. Weber K. Rear-facing restraint for small child passengers—a medical alert. *Univ Mich Transportation Res Inst Res Rev*. 1995;25:12–17
9. American Academy of Pediatrics. Transporting children with special needs. *AAP Safe Ride News Insert*. 1993;Winter
10. American Academy of Pediatrics. *Child Restraint Systems: Getting It Right*. Speaker's and resource kit. Elk Grove Village, IL: American Academy of Pediatrics. In press

# AMERICAN ACADEMY OF PEDIATRICS

# Screening Infants and Young Children for Developmental Disabilities

Committee on Children With Disabilities    (RE9414)

Early identification of children with developmental disabilities leads to effective therapy of conditions for which definitive treatment is available. However, even in those instances in which the condition cannot be fully reversed, early intervention improves children's outcomes and enables families to develop the strategies and obtain the resources for successful family functioning. Much of the impact of early intervention results from fostering a more comfortable and developmentally appropriate interaction between the parents and their child with a disability.

## DEFINITION

Screening is a "brief assessment procedure designed to identify children who should receive more intensive diagnosis or assessment."[1] Early childhood developmental screening does not consist of administering a single instrument at one point in time, but rather is a set of processes and procedures used over time. The following guidelines are recommended by the Task Force on Screening and Assessment of the National Early Childhood Technical Assistance System[1]:

- Screening should be viewed as a service and part of the intervention process.
- Screening processes, procedures, and instruments should only be used for their intended purpose.
- Multiple sources of information should be utilized.
- Screening should be performed on a recurrent or periodic basis.
- Screening should be viewed as only one path to further assessment and the acquisition of services, with social and medical risk factors also being considered in decisions about evaluation and intervention.
- Procedures should be reliable and valid.
- Family members should be included as part of the process.
- Screening is more effective when familiar tasks and settings are used.
- Procedures must be culturally sensitive.
- Screening should be performed by individuals with training in the procedures.

Screening does not measure a child's intelligence quotient, rather it is aimed at identifying those children who may need more comprehensive evaluations. Such evaluations may lead to the development of an interdisciplinary comprehensive plan of remediation for a child with a disability, to a realization that there is no significant problem, or to a decision that further observation is warranted.[1] The act of screening also serves the purpose of clearly communicating to parents the pediatrician's interest in the development as well as the physical health of the child.[2] If appropriate, the pediatrician should foster awareness and acceptance of the possible developmental disability.

Public Law 99-457 (reauthorized as Pub L 102-119, The Individuals with Disabilities Education Act)[3] mandates early identification of, and intervention for, developmental disabilities. Since the passage of that law, the emphasis in screening has shifted to a younger age, with the current focus being on infants and children birth through 2 years of age.[3] This is an age at which the pediatrician is very closely involved with children and families and is in a position to have significant impact on the course of the child's development. Public Law 99-457 and The Individuals with Disabilities Education Act have also led to the development of community systems for tracking of high-risk infants and resources for referring infants and young children for intervention. The emphasis on earlier identification creates the opportunity to provide the benefits of early intervention, but also poses greater challenges in the sphere of screening. Parents expect their pediatricians to give them guidance on developmental issues, but will turn to other community systems if the pediatrician does not fill this role. Children and families are best served when pediatricians' screening efforts are coordinated with the tracking and intervention services available in the community.

## ISSUES IN METHODOLOGY

Delays or deviations in development may come to the attention of professionals and parents because the child is known to have risk factors by history, has physical findings or medical conditions likely to be associated with delays, or manifests delays at the time of observation. The first two factors are as useful in a very young child as in an older one, but some developmental delays are more difficult to assess early. A delay in a skill becomes evident only at the age when that developmental milestone is expected. For example, motor skills, which change rapidly in the first 2 years, are the easiest milestones to observe, but are the least predictive for future intelligence. Language skills are usually identified later but are better predictors of future intelligence and school performance.[4]

Developmental disabilities encompass a spectrum of problems of varying kinds and severity. Although broad agreement exists as to what constitutes clear-cut delay or deviation, there is not complete consensus among professionals, or between parents and physicians, as to the severity at which evaluation and intervention become appropriate and when deviations from norms are sufficient to warrant further clinical attention. The central dilemma for the pediatrician who screens patients is that identification must precede services, and the act of identifying a child as one who needs further assessment for developmental disabilities provokes anxiety in parents. This concern may create a tendency to identify only markedly delayed children, denying other children potential access to needed care.

The limited ability of infant tests, whether intended for screening or definitive diagnosis of intellectual functioning, to predict future function has led to controversy concerning their use. However, when physicians use only clinical impressions, estimates of children's developmental status are often inaccurate.[5] The advantage of screening instruments is that they state their norms explicitly, serve as a reminder to the pediatrician to observe development, and are an efficient way to record the observations.

The Denver-II, which is a successor to the Denver Developmental Screening Test, is a brief, validated test with which many pediatricians are familiar.[6] Although it has been criticized for having limited specificity and therefore risks overreferring, it has high rates of sensitivity and identifies delayed children correctly in a high proportion of cases.[7] Because the Denver II is intended to be used in the context of a process that includes other sources of information and multiple points in time, it is a useful part of the screening. The Early Language Milestones is another instrument suitable for office screening that was designed for identifying delays in language in children less than 3 years of age.[8] A recent review of commonly used screening instruments is available.[1] Although there is still a paucity of adequately validated tests that are brief and can be used for infants, the growing interest in assessment of infants and young children will likely result in the development of new instruments and methods.

Because the screening process selects those children who will receive the benefits of more intensive evaluation or of treatment after evaluation, all children should be screened for developmental disabilities. Screening is not the same as evaluation, diagnosis, or planning of treatment and represents the first step leading to a multidisciplinary evaluation. In the optimal situation, each child should have a defined medical home for primary care, and screening procedures should be incorporated into the ongoing health care of the child.

## SCREENING PROCESS

Essential components of the screening process are as follows:

- Sensitive attention to parental concerns
- Thoughtful inquiry about parental observations
- Observation of a wide variety of the child's behaviors

- Examination of specific developmental attainments
- Use of all encounters for observing and recording developmental status
- Screening of vision and hearing to rule out sensory impairment as a cause of the delay
- Observation of parent-child interaction.

## REQUIRED SKILLS AND PROCEDURES

To screen for developmental disabilities and intervene with the identified children and their families, the primary pediatrician must have the clinical skills and institute the procedures listed below:

1. Maintain and update her or his knowledge about developmental issues, risk factors, screening techniques, and community resources for consultation and intervention
2. Acquire skills in the administration and interpretation of a formal developmental screening technique
3. Develop a strategy to provide periodic screening in the context of office-based primary care, including the following:
   - Developmental screening of all children in the practice
   - Recognizing abnormal appearance and function during health care maintenance examinations
   - Recognizing high-risk medical and environmental situations while taking routine medical and social histories
   - Actively seeking observations and concerns from parents about their child's development
   - Recognizing troubled parent-child interaction from history or observation
   - Performing periodic rescreenings of practice populations to discover the possible emergence of new risk situations or the child's difficulty in meeting more advanced developmental expectations
4. Maintain updated information on existing community resources for serving infants and children at risk for, or with, developmental delays and their families;
5. Maintain linkages with these resources and coordinate patient care with them;
6. Increase parents' awareness of developmental disabilities and of resources for intervention by such methods as display and distribution of educational materials in the office; and
7. Be available to families to interpret consultants' findings.

Ongoing involvement with the family permits the pediatrician to respond to parental concerns about the child's development when such concerns exist. When parents are not aware of a delay that is present, the pediatrician can guide them toward closer observation of their child and thus enable them to recognize the delay. Referral for evaluation and services can take place only after the pediatrician has succeeded in this challenging task. At that point the pediatrician's role shifts to one of involvement in the evaluation as appropriate, referral to available community resources for intervention and family support, assistance in understanding the evaluation results, assessment and coordination of services, and monitoring the child's developmental progress as part of the ongoing pediatric care.

## CONCLUSION

Early identification of children with developmental disabilities can lead to treatment or amelioration of the severity of a disability and its impact on the functioning of the child and family. Because developmental screening is a process that selects those children who will receive the benefits of more intensive evaluation, or of treatment, all infants and children should be screened for developmental disabilities, otherwise some may be denied access to needed care. Successful early identification of developmental disabilities requires the pediatrician to be skilled in the use of screening techniques and of developmental surveillance, to actively seek parental concerns about development, and to create linkages with available resources in the community. Because community systems vary from one locality to another and may change over time, the physician's information must be updated on a regular basis. Children and families are best served when the primary pediatrician providing health supervision services collaborates with the tracking and intervention services available in the community.

COMMITTEE ON CHILDREN WITH DISABILITIES, 1993 to 1994
James Perrin, MD, Chair
Gerald Erenberg, MD
Ruth K. Kaminer, MD
Robert La Camera, MD
John A. Nackashi, MD
John R. Poncher, MD
Virginia Randall, MD

Renee C. Wachtel, MD
Philip R. Ziring, MD

LIAISON REPRESENTATIVES
Connie Garner, RN, MSN, EdD, US Dept of Education Programs
Debbie Gaebler, MD, American Academy of Physical Medicine and Rehabilitation
Joseph G. Hollowell, MD, Center for Disease Control and Center for Environmental Health and Injury Control
Merle McPherson, MD, Maternal and Child Health Bureau, Dept of Health & Human Services

SECTION LIAISON
Harry Gewanter, MD, Section on Rheumatology

CONSULTANT
Avrum Katcher, MD

## REFERENCES

1. Meisels SJ, Provence S. *Screening Assessment. Guidelines for Identifying Young Disabled and Developmentally Vulnerable Children and Their Families.* Washington, DC: Zero to Three/National Center for Clinical Infant Programs; 1989
2. Kaminer R, Jedrysek E. Early identification of developmental disabilities. *Pediatr Ann.* 1982;11:427–437
3. Individuals With Disabilities Education Act of 1991 (Pub L No. 102–119)
4. Stevenson J. Predictive value of speech and language screening. *Dev Med Child Neurol.* 1984;26:528–538
5. Dworkin PH. Developmental screening: still expecting the impossible? *Pediatrics.* 1992;89:1253–1255
6. Frankenburg WK, Dodds J, Archer P, Shapiro H, Bresnick B. *Denver-II Screening Manual.* Denver, CO: Denver Developmental Materials, Inc; 1990
7. Glascoe FP, Byrne KE, Ashford LG, Johnson KL, Chang B, Strickland B. Accuracy of the Denver-II in developmental screening. *Pediatrics.* 1992; 89:1221–1225
8. Coplan J, Gleason JR, Ryan R, Burke MG, Williams ML. Validation of an early language milestone scale in a high-risk population. *Pediatrics.* 1982;70:677–683

# AMERICAN ACADEMY OF PEDIATRICS

## Transition of Care Provided for Adolescents With Special Health Care Needs (RE9645)

Committee on Children With Disabilities and Committee on Adolescence

ABSTRACT. This policy statement describes how the pediatrician can work closely with patients with special health care needs and their families as an advocate and educator to help them adapt positively to an adult-focused system of health care. Issues in health care transitions including independence and dependence, education and vocational issues, insurance issues and limitations, Social Security, and hospitalization are outlined.

Families with children with chronic illness, cognitive or sensory impairment, physical disabilities, and/or other special health care needs often face a particularly difficult transition from adolescent to adult health care.

## BACKGROUND

During the past two decades, the survival rates associated with most chronic illnesses have improved greatly such that more than 90% of children with a chronic illness and/or disability now survive to adulthood.[1]

Improved understanding of prevention and treatment (including better nutrition, anti-inflammatory and antimicrobial agents, enzyme replacement therapy, and earlier multidisciplinary interventions for many conditions) has resulted in successful therapeutic interventions that diminish long-term or secondary disability and improve long-term function. For example, children and adults who require mechanical ventilation or oxygen therapy not only survive but also can attend school and obtain employment. Societal changes now encourage more children and adults with substantial cognitive and/or physical impairments to live at home or in community settings with appropriate support.[2]

Most chronically ill and/or disabled individuals want to live full, productive lives. Pediatricians can play a critical role in reinforcing positive attitudes and beliefs while helping adolescents and their families to make appropriate transitions to adult health care. Some young adults will require ongoing medical care for chronic health conditions (eg, diabetes,

arthritis, and severe asthma), whereas others may require technological assistance (eg, ventilation, specialized wheelchairs, or communication devices) or personal care attendants. Still others, especially those young adults with primarily developmental disabilities, may need only supported living assistance (eg, specialized housing or supportive employment).

The pediatrician (or other health care providers who may be providing a medical home for children and adolescents with disabilities) should play a central role in helping adolescents and their families make the transition to adult health care. Toward this end, the pediatrician needs to know which practitioners in the community have the clinical skills needed and an interest in working with adults with disabilities.

Under some circumstances, young adults with special health care needs may choose to continue with their current health care supervision because some pediatricians comfortable with adult health and sexuality issues can provide adult-oriented medical care if the patient and family agree. Criteria and timing for eventual transitions will vary.

## ISSUES IN HEALTH CARE TRANSITIONS

Most adolescents with chronic conditions require coordinated care that frequently involves multiple health care providers. Coordination and access may be more difficult when adolescents reach adulthood; often, an entirely new group of health care providers assume responsibility for adult patients. These providers may be unfamiliar with the patients' histories and the priorities and concerns of these patients and their families.[3]

Also, adolescents with special health care needs may need to adjust to the possible loss of a close and longstanding relationship with their pediatrician and other specialists when transferring to adult health care. This change may be difficult, because many pediatricians often work with multidisciplinary teams while adult-oriented health care providers tend to focus more on specific system-oriented complaints and rely on independent consultants for further specialty care. Because many adult health care providers receive only limited training regarding adolescent or young adult disorders associated with disabilities and transitional issues, the provider may be unfamiliar with the disabling condition (eg, cystic fibrosis or spina bifida) and its management.

Schidlow and Fiel have summarized other major

obstacles to smooth transitions from adolescent to adult health care. The severity of the illness or disability, the level of maturity, acceptance and understanding of the patient, additional environmental or family stresses, the need for control by parents or health care provider, a distorted perception (by parents or health care provider) of potential patient outcomes, and lack of patient or family support systems all may contribute to transition stress.

### Independence and Dependence

The goal for all children is to move progressively from complete dependence toward independence. Children with disabilities, regardless of cause, should be encouraged to develop the highest possible level of independence based on a realistic and objective evaluation of their abilities and limitations. The adolescent and the family may be unsure of the benefits of greater independence or even unaware of the patient's ability to achieve partial or total independence.[4]

The typically healthy desire for independence may be misconstrued by some adolescents with diabetes as license to avoid administering insulin regularly but may help the youth with cerebral palsy who, despite parental or physician protests, decides to use a wheelchair instead of crutches to participate with peers more actively.

For adolescents who are more dependent on others for a variety of care needs, the acquisition of some of the skills needed for self-care and independent living can contribute to a more successful and comfortable life at home or preparation for group homes or other adult living arrangements. This learning promotes self-esteem and facilitates more full participation in their community. Toward this end, the person with a disability should have the opportunity to acquire skills to understand and to develop a sense of financial responsibility when appropriate.

The development of skills for independent living (such as living alone or in assisted-living accommodations, planning or preparing meals, or grocery shopping) frequently requires assistance from multiple disciplines. The pediatrician can assist in the planning process by informing the patient, family, and others involved in training about the patient's special health care needs, and by providing clear and specific recommendations regarding the abilities of the patient and the possible need to alter the environment.

### Education and Vocational Issues

Most adolescents with disabilities have participated in modified educational programs. Frequent and prolonged hospitalizations or illness convalescence can interrupt continuity or delay the achievement of educational goals. Many well-intentioned programs offer limited opportunities for experiences outside the school and may fail to prepare the adolescent for many life experiences and the world of work and independent living.[5]

Preparation for vocational assessment and training should not be postponed until the student is 18 to 21 years old because training may be prolonged for the adolescent with a disability. The pediatrician can assist the adolescent, family, and school to understand the medical aspects of the student's condition and seek an appropriate person to coordinate the evaluation and transition to higher education or vocational training.[6-8]

The pediatrician should be aware that the nationwide federal/state vocational rehabilitation program has an agency in each state capital as well as other local offices. These locations can be found in the telephone directory (under the state listing for Rehabilitative Services or Vocational Rehabilitation Services.) These agencies assist eligible people with disabilities to define a suitable employment goal, assist with additional educational opportunities, and assist with employment. Supported or sheltered employment options provide opportunities that can enhance the quality of life and personal satisfaction of young people with severe disabilities.[9] The Americans With Disabilities Act also has the potential to help with issues of access to job opportunities and public facilities.[10]

### Insurance Issues and Limitations

Adolescents with chronic illnesses and disabilities face special problems regarding access to health insurance, especially when they are no longer covered by their parents' insurance.[11,12] Currently, insurance provisions regarding preexisting medical conditions may limit or even preclude insurance eligibility for many. Insurance coverage for therapies important to the disabled person's mobility, communication, or physical and psychological functioning often are not provided or provided only for a very limited number of hours per year if they are covered.

The adolescent or young adult with disabilities often requires insurance that covers a broad range of services, including multiple medical specialty consultations, laboratory tests, equipment, and prescription plans.[13] Such insurance rarely is available to many workers with disabilities which may limit their productivity on the job or the types of jobs for which they are qualified, forcing them to accept lower-wage employment that may not offer insurance or provide the types of benefits needed at an affordable cost.

### Social Security

The Social Security Administration directs two programs of financial assistance to eligible persons during the transition process.[14,15]

First, the Supplemental Security Income program provides cash benefits for low-income persons who are blind or have other disabilities. Recent Supplemental Security Income changes help children and those younger than 18 years with disabilities to qualify for benefits. Persons older than 18 years are eligible to receive monthly payments if they have little or no income or resources (eg, a savings account) and have a substantial disability.

Second, the Social Security Disability Income considers the employment status of the applicant's parents. "Benefits are paid to persons who become disabled before age 22 if at least one of their parents had worked a certain amount of time under Social Security but now is disabled, retired, and/or deceased."

Recent legislation has made major changes in both programs to encourage people with disabilities receiving these benefits to work and to become independent. Also, certain provisions of Supplemental Security Income allow for the maintenance of Medicaid coverage even when the young adult becomes employed.[16]

Information is available through the local Social Security office or by calling the Social Security Administration toll free at 1–800–772–1213 (voice) or 1–800–325–0778 (TDD).

### Hospitalization

Young adults with a chronic disease or special health care needs may require frequent hospitalization, just as they did during childhood. As they mature, many develop ambivalent feelings regarding hospitalization, particularly when they become the oldest patients in the pediatric or adolescent unit. At the same time, however, their familiarity and comfort with the unit personnel, policies, and procedures may make them reluctant to enter an adult unit.

Inpatient care should be a part of the short- and long-term planning for management of the adolescent and young adult with special health care needs. Hospitalization may be an essential or infrequent adjunct to a health care program but still is subject to issues of transition and planning. Preferably, arrangements for hospital care should not be made on an urgent or emergent basis but planned well in advance with attention to detail.

The individual plan for hospitalization should consider whether the adolescent or young adult prefers admission to an adolescent or adult unit. It is important that the unit staff receive training in the management of those long-term conditions that arise during childhood or adolescence. When pediatricians continue to provide primary care for young adult patients, they should seek admitting privileges to the adult unit to ensure their continuing participation as the primary attending physician or as a consultant.

## SUMMARY AND RECOMMENDATIONS

Technical advances and improved care for children with chronic diseases have allowed most children with chronic disabilities to reach adulthood. Planning is essential to achieve appropriate transition from pediatric health care to adult health care. Transition planning should:

- begin early, with special attention to maximizing opportunities for independence and for the necessary health, educational, and social services;
- include active participation of the family and patient in the process;
- consider the patient individually, realistically, and positively, encouraging functional independence and appropriate attitudes toward self-worth and interpersonal relationships (including issues of sexuality);
- encourage the patient's willingness or ability to accept the plan;
- consider having the pediatrician and the adult health care practitioner as comanagers for a period of time (eg, 1 or 2 years); and include recommendations by the pediatrician for referral to adult health care providers (especially subspecialists) who are sensitive to and have an interest in families that include adults with special health care needs.

The pediatrician should participate actively in the above process and become aware of local, state, and national resources for family and patient assistance (eg, Vocational Rehabilitation Services and Social Security Administration) and, if necessary, help patients and their families gain access to the appropriate agencies or information.

Above all, the pediatrician should work closely with patients and their families as advocate and educator to help them adapt positively to an adult-focused system of health care.

SECTION LIAISON
Samuel Leavitt, MD
    Section on School Health

CONSULTANT
Donald Greydanus, MD

## REFERENCES

1. Bronheim S, Fiel S, Schidlow D, Magrab P, Boczar K, Dillon C. *Crossings: A Manual for Transition of Chronically Ill Youth to Adult Health Care.* Washington, DC: Georgetown University Child Development Center;

2. Gortmaker SL, Perrin JM, Weitzman M, Homer CJ, Sobol AM. An unexpected success story: transition to adulthood in youth with chronic physical health conditions. *J Res Adolesc.* 1993;3:317–336

3. Schidlow D, Fiel B. Life beyond pediatrics: transition of chronically ill adolescents from pediatrics to adult health care systems. *Med Clin North Am.* 1990;74:1113–1120

4. Pless IB, Power C, Peckham CS. Long-term psychological sequelae of chronic physical disorders in childhood. *Pediatrics.* 1993;91:1131–1136

5. Wehman P, Moon MS, Everson JM, Wood W, Barcus JM. *Transition From School to Work: New Challenges for Youth With Severe Disabilities.* Baltimore, MD: Paul H. Brooks Publishing Co; 1988

6. Harris L and Associates, Inc. *The ICD Survey of Disabled Americans: Bringing Disabled Americans into the Mainstream, a Nationwide Survey of 1000 Disabled People.* New York, NY: International Center for the Disabled; 1986

7. *Options After High School for Youth With Disabilities.* Washington, DC: NICHY Transition Summary. National Information Center for Children and Youth With Disabilities; 1991:7

8. Kiernan WE, Brinkman L. Barriers to employment for adults with developmental disabilities. In: Kiernan WE, Stark JA, eds. *Employment Options for Adults With Developmental Disabilities.* Logan, UT: Utah State University Affiliated Facility, Developmental Center for Handicapped Persons; 1985:160–174

9. Wehman P, Moon MS. *Vocational Rehabilitation and Supported Employment.* Baltimore, MD: Paul H. Brookes Publishing Co; 1988

10. Amendments to the Rehabilitation Act, Pub L No. 99–506(1986)

11. Newacheck PW. Adolescents with special health needs: prevalence, severity, and access to health services. *Pediatrics.* 1989;84:872–881

12. Newacheck PW, McManus MA. Health insurance status of adolescents in the United States. *Pediatrics.* 1989;84:699–708

13. Perrin JM. Health care reform and the special needs of children. *Pediatrics.* 1994;93:504–506

14. Magrab PR, Millar HEC. *Surgeon General's Conference: Growing Up and Getting Medical Care: Youth With Special Health Care Needs.* Washington, DC: The Bureau of Maternal and Child Health and Resources Development; 1989

15. *SSI: New Opportunities for Children With Disabilities.* Washington, DC: Mental Health Law Project; 1995

16. Perrin JM, Stein RE. Reinterpreting disability: changes in Supplemental Security Income for Children. *Pediatrics.* 1991;88:1047–1051

## SUGGESTED READINGS

Blum RW. The disabled adolescent: an orientation. In: Hofmann A, Greydanus D, eds. *Adolescent Medicine.* East Norwalk, CT: Appleton & Lange; 1989

Capelli M, MacDonald NE, McGrath PJ. Assessment of readiness to transfer to adult care for adolescents with cystic fibrosis. *Child Health Care.* 1989; 18:218–224

Rettig P, Athreya BH. Adolescents with chronic disease: transition to adult health care. *Arthritis Care Res.* 1991;4:174–180

# RELATED ARTICLES

# STRATEGIES FOR MANAGED CARE
## An Update from the Committee on Child Health Financing

# MANAGED CARE AND CHILDREN WITH SPECIAL HEALTH CARE NEEDS: CREATING A MEDICAL HOME

Managed care occupies an increasingly prominent position in today's health care environment. Traditional non-managed indemnity plans now represent only 35 percent of insurance coverage. Managed care penetration in some states has risen as high as 35 to 40 percent, and 19 states have applied for or been granted waivers to develop managed care programs for their Medicaid-eligible population.

Few pediatricians in practice remain untouched by the rapid shifts in payment mechanisms, the insurer's goal of curbing utilization and reducing costs, and newly formed networks of specialists and hospitals. A recent AAP Department of Research periodic survey discovered that in 1993, 64.2 percent of AAP members providing ambulatory care said that at least half of their insured patients are in managed care. Nearly one-fourth (23.7 percent) of pediatricians said 90 to 100 percent of their patients are in managed care.

While the payment environment shifts to managed care, significant changes also have occurred in the shape of pediatrics itself. Advances in medicine and surgery have improved life expectancies for children with a wide variety of chronic illnesses and disabilities. These same advances have created new outpatient options for much of the care for both chronic and acute conditions. Yet there has been difficulty in developing a standard definition of "children with special health care needs," and thus identifying the size of this population. Current estimates are that 15 to 20 million children have some kind of chronic condition. Severe health conditions that are likely to require extensive daily caretaking affect between 1 million and 2 million youngsters. However, the definitions that have been developed tend to have a broader focus than just chronic conditions. For example, one of the many working definitions states, "Children with special health care needs are those who have or are at increased risk for chronic physical,

developmental, behavioral, or emotional conditions and who also require health and related services of a type and amount beyond that required by children generally."

Children with special health care needs have a broad range of primary, specialized, and related service requirements. In addition to well child care, health promotion, and disease prevention, children with special health care needs often require specialty care, diagnostic and intervention strategies, home therapies, and ongoing ancillary services, such as occupational therapy, physical therapy, speech therapy, and individual and family counseling, as well as the long-term management of ongoing medical complications. Many of these children also depend on health care services at home, in school, and in the community. Recognizing that children with chronic conditions have these needs, managed care systems face a critical issue: can they control utilization and still offer the full range of appropriate services?

This question taps inherent tensions. Managed care plans, in striving to control costs, may or may not include the broad range of service options in the benefit packages necessary for children with chronic illness. Even if the managed care system has contractual language to cover needed services, the route to establish medical necessity may be complex, prolonged, and controlled by non-pediatric decision makers. In addition, the risk of caring for children with chronic conditions is not well-defined and is subject to unexpected and frequent changes of care plans with potentially costly additions. Given these challenges, it is critical to explore the role of pediatricians in the managed care environment as they work to balance the provision of comprehensive, quality health care with the demands to manage service utilization among children with special health care needs.

## How Primary Care Physicians Fit

Managed care means accountability for the health care dollar. Utilization is closely monitored to avoid unnecessary duplication of service, unwarranted emergency room use, specialty referrals, and the use of out-of-network services.

Managed care can mean a tight surveillance of physician decision making regarding referrals, as well as the use of laboratory tests and ancillary services. Such surveillance quickly leads to provider frustration. Physicians find their health delivery options constrained and their medical judgment overruled. When health care plans monitor utilization and access to health care services solely to control costs, the delivery of quality health care may be in jeopardy.

By contrast, if managed care puts the keys in the hands of the provider to open and monitor the delivery of services through gatekeeping, an appropriate system of care is possible. Under the best of circumstances, the keys open the door to the medical home where the patient's family and provider work together to assure that services are family-centered, coordinated, and comprehensive. Only time will tell how often this model of care is achieved. The following sections outline the components of a successful medical home model for children with special health care needs.

Children with special health care needs demand a great deal from pediatric primary health care providers. Opening the door to the medical home requires specific well-honed skills to meet utilization and budgetary constraints imposed by managed care. Providers do best when they are able to manage their own time, ensure the appropriate flow of resources, and when they feel confident about how to deal with a wide range of medical problems.

*Specific skills*: To create an effective medical home, the primary care physician should establish a partnership with the child's family. The AAP policy statement on the Medical Home provides a definition of "medical home."

Together, the primary care physician and the family should develop a long-range health care plan for the child. This plan should anticipate infancy, early and middle childhood, and adolescent issues, and should encompass the medical, developmental, educational, and social issues that are commonly encountered by children with chronic health conditions.

By collaborating with the family on the child's care plan, the primary care physician can work toward optimal utilization of necessary services. Intervention points should be mapped out to clarify which specialists should be involved, why they are needed, and the amount of time for which they are needed. The primary care pediatrician should educate the managed care plan about the necessity for referrals to pediatric medical subspecialists and surgical specialists and the need for the primary care physician to serve as the coordinator of all care that will be provided. In addition, since education is paramount for children with special health care needs, pediatricians should also work with managed care plans to promote a relationship between the managed care plan and school-based or school-linked health care centers. Having such a conduit improves the family's access to critical information and ensures a central repository for the medical record. It also cuts down on the expensive physician shopping that so often results in duplication of effort and exhaustive evaluations.

To serve as the medical home, the primary care pediatrician needs a reliable network of pediatric medical subspecialists and surgical specialists available in the managed care system who can evaluate the patient and communicate their findings promptly and completely. Two issues continue to hamper this function in managed care systems. First, primary and specialty care pediatricians are most familiar with a fee-for-service world where such communication holds much less value. Managed care incentives are changing old patterns of behavior, but there is still a lot of progress to be made. The second problem is that some managed care systems see children as "little adults." They do not recognize the unique medical, developmental, and social concerns of children and the importance of referral to pediatric medical subspecialists and surgical specialists. As a result, some physicians working in managed care have found themselves severely constrained in their choice of specialists. Creating a medical home in managed care will require strong advocacy for the development of a network of pediatric medical subspecialists, pediatric surgical specialists and consultants as part of each managed care organization. It is incumbent upon the pediatrician entering a managed care contract to review the plan's provider list to determine the extent to which pediatric medical subspecialists and surgical specialists are part of the network. If a certain specialist is not part of the network, open a line of communication to the plan and document the reason why a child with certain conditions should be seen by this particular specialist. It is also important to educate families about the managed care plan's service coverage and prior authorization policies and convince them that they too should communicate their concerns to the managed care plan if problems arise.

Pediatricians should also work with managed care plans to assure that the array of services offered are pediatric in their orientation and that families can access these services without a major hassle. Managed care plans may assume that other state public health programs will fill the gaps, especially for Medicaid-enrolled children. Once again, pediatricians must become advocates for their patients and work with the managed care plans to ensure that both the array and focus of the services are pediatric-oriented.

*Time:* Caring for children with special health care needs takes more time than caring for their healthier peers. Their histories are longer and their physical examinations reveal more findings. Children who are developmentally disabled require different techniques for engagement with the provider to elicit the necessary information. Moreover, it takes time to coordinate subspecialty referrals and hospitalizations, document the medical record appropriately, and complete necessary forms. Communicating with home care companies, school nurses, and other community-based agencies also requires a significant amount of time. As a result, the pediatrician in practice who has agreed to manage the care of a panel of patients with chronic illness needs to factor that time into the workday and into any arrangements made with partners and clinical co-workers. It is critical to document the time spent with these patients. Documentation is a key defense, especially in this era of physician profiling.

*Reimbursement:* One way to protect the time for managing the care of children with special health care needs is to negotiate an enhanced capitation rate for caring for such children. To offer a medical home to a number of such children in their panel, the pediatrician should negotiate a favorable capitation rate with the managed care organization in advance. The capitation rate should include the complexity of coordinating activities as well as the increased time associated with face-to-face encounters. When making the case for an enhanced capitation rate, it is most helpful to have a clear idea of the number of children involved as well as the services they are likely to require. This is where documentation is important. Data on the covered population can be obtained from the managed care plan or the employer. Clinical pathways and practice guidelines offer valuable new resources to project needed resources. Always check with your managed care plan to determine the guidelines that are used and how they are used. If children are covered under Medicaid, it is important to ensure that the capitation rate reflects the full range of required benefits such as Early and Periodic Screening, Diagnosis, and Treatment (EPSDT).

A major concern for primary care physicians is the burden that risk-sharing arrangements may place on them. Partially and fully capitated reimbursement strategies can put the physician at risk for specialty referrals and other medically necessary, expensive ancillary services. Individual physicians should avoid accepting risk for all physician services. If physicians are to take risk, it should be at the medical group or IPA level (usually all physicians, but at least all primary care physicians). Ideally, an appropriate capitation rate adjusted for case-mix or severity should be negotiated with the insurer. Some managed care plans have adopted the Ambulatory Care Group (ACG) system developed by Johns Hopkins University. ACGs provide a method to compare costs to diagnoses in a known population. However, there is limited experience of using the ACGs in the pediatric population. ACGs work as follows:

1. Each patient in a population is assigned to a particular ACG depending upon a relatively complicated analysis of all diagnoses associated with each patient.

2. The capitation rate for each ACG in the population is calculated by summing the costs for all patients in that ACG and dividing by the number of patients assigned to that ACG.

3. The capitation rate for each ACG in this population is compared to the capitation rate for each ACG from a population with similar characteristics to mathematically evaluate the cost-efficiency of particular providers. This is a risk-adjusted comparison.

A 1995 Physician Payment Review Commission (PPRC) report highlighting the type of arrangements managed care plans make with physicians discovered that less than one-fifth of plans (group/staff and network/IPA models) use a health status adjuster to the physician capitation rate. For the most part, the capitation adjustments are based on demographic data. Network/IPA models use a health status risk adjuster more than group/staff models. Although the study only involved 80 plans, it does illustrate how infrequent health status is used to adjust capitation rates. Until better data are available on the appropriate capitation rates for children with complex medical and developmental needs, physicians should consider whether or not to purchase reinsurance with stop-loss provisions.

Primary care providers who work to establish a medical home for children with special health care needs may encounter other frustrations, specifically their limitations in deciding how the capitated dollar is allocated. Given a fixed amount of money, who chooses whether the dollars are spent on primary versus specialty care, inpatient versus outpatient services, or renting versus buying equipment? How radical can the solutions be? Can a family member or neighbor be paid to deliver home care services, thus saving nursing care dollars? Around the country, groups of health care policy experts are exploring such options under the auspices of the Robert Wood Johnson Foundation, the Annie E. Casey Foundation, the Packard Foundation, the Pew Charitable Trust, the federal Maternal and Child Health Bureau (MCHB), the Health Care Financing Administration (HCFA), and others concerned about balancing the cost and service requirements of children with special health care needs. New projects are underway to examine pediatric risk adjustment models, quality of care measures for chronic childhood illness, pediatric managed care models and innovations, and more.

To provide adequate care for children with special health care needs, it is often necessary to tap other monetary sources—the state Medicaid program, the Title V Maternal & Child Health Program, Supplemental Security Income (SSI), Part B and Part H of the Individuals with Disabilities Education Act, and children's mental health programs. These funding sources can sometimes help with home care, ancillary services, and family support. Unfortunately, it often takes families and their physicians an inordinate amount of time to learn about these resources and about the children's eligibility to receive these dollars. Some managed care plans are unaware of these resources; therefore, pediatricians may want to take the initiative and educate them on these options. Centralization of this information benefits the patient, family, provider, and plan.

*Medical management:* In pediatrics, an ongoing challenge for primary care physicians is the fact that while few children have severe chronic conditions and disabilities, there are many different causes of the conditions—congenital, infectious, traumatic, oncologic—and each specific condition may require a different management strategy. In part, it is the diverse nature of childhood chronic illness that has engendered the development of the many specialties and subspecialties. Pediatricians managing the care of children with special health care needs should have a strong

network of pediatric medical subspecialists, pediatric surgical specialists, and consultants. Unfortunately, however, many managed care networks have a limited pediatric specialist network and rely on adult specialists who may be unfamiliar with the intricacies of the care of children with special health care needs. One single pediatrician cannot possibly know all the diagnostic, management, and treatment requirements for every chronic illness he or she may encounter over the course of practice, but there are certain underlying principles of chronic care management that are generic. The following principles allow effective co-management between primary care physicians and pediatric specialists.

1. A diagnosis and prognosis should be established, realizing that this is not always possible or cost-effective.

2. In the absence of an etiologic diagnosis, it is helpful to families to have as full an explanation of symptoms and function as possible and a forthright plan for dealing with uncertainty.

3. Once a diagnosis or characterization of the problem is established, functional/developmental abilities should be determined. It is also helpful to determine the medical, surgical, habilitative, and rehabilitative or maintenance interventions that are currently recommended and available for the child's condition.

4. The risks and benefits of each intervention need to be explored and pursued together with the child's family. These risks may include family burden as well as medical and psychosocial risks for the child.

5. Referral to appropriate specialists does not mean that care of the patient is relinquished by the primary care provider, which in some cases may be quite appropriate; however, confusion occurs if the transfer of the primary care responsibility is not made explicit. The best system is co-management with the use of clearly delineated care protocols.

## The Role of Specialists in Managed Care

Specialty care is also affected by the new managed care arrangements. On one hand, pediatric medical subspecialists, pediatric surgical specialists, and hospitals can count on a referral base from the managed care alliances they make. On the other hand, these pediatric specialists may have an increasingly difficult time attracting patients because of preferred provider arrangements. Moreover, as managed care plans strive to constrain utilization, they may tend to use adult specialists.

For managed care to work for children with special health care needs, effective communication systems are essential. To the extent that primary care and specialty providers can share a common data-base that includes pertinent history, physical examination, laboratory, and radiologic information, care can be streamlined and coordinated. Open and timely communication between the primary care physician and specialists should result in appropriate management of problems and elimination of unnecessary referrals.

In a well-defined or organized system, the primary care provider serves as the coordinator of all care provided. In this role, the pediatrician obtains all the initial data before referring the child to the specialist. The pediatric medical subspecialist or surgical specialist can then proceed to evaluate the need for specialized procedures and interventions, provide the necessary care, and communicate with the primary care physician. Such a system works when pediatric medical subspecialists, pediatric surgical specialists, and primary care pediatricians can spend some of their time educating each other about the need for communication of complete clinical information regarding the referral and after-care. Patient-specific communication is best done on a one-to-one basis. More generic education about care coordination/case management takes place at hospital grand rounds, pediatric society meetings, and continuing medical education (CME) courses. Increasingly, these courses are being sponsored by the managed care programs themselves. As new house officers and fellows take part in training programs, there will need to be increased emphasis on the specialist-generalist co-management paradigms.

## Steps to Meet the Challenge

There is no question that fitting children with special health care needs into managed care is a challenge, but several steps should improve the chances for success:

1. Define the population of children you are seeing who have special health care needs. To characterize the children with more complex needs, several alternatives are available. If the managed care company uses ICD-9 codes, you can request a computer printout for children with codes covering chronic illness and disabilities. Another way of capturing the children with complex conditions in your panel is to ask for a computer printout of hospitalizations and select the group of children with the most frequent, highest cost, and longest stays. This initial step of defining the population will give a sense of the work that is needed, targets for decreasing utilization, and information for negotiating an enhanced capitation rate.

2. Work with the utilization management and quality of care staff in the managed care organization to create a shared data-base between primary care and specialist physicians, the emergency department, and the hospital(s). This will capitalize on the major benefit of network development, reduce duplicate work, and improve patient care.

3. With each patient and family, define the extent of the health and functional needs based on the diagnosis, condition, and resources at home and in the community. Creating such a yardstick helps with both short-term and long-term goals and may serve as a basis for a care pathway that can be approved by the managed care plan.

4. Create a health care plan together with the family and the child's other providers that is approved by the managed care plan. Outline the efforts to be made to cut down on duplication of effort and establish improved communication. Monitor the health care plan on a periodic basis to help ensure that the child indeed has a medical home.

5. Work with the quality of care staff of the managed care plan to develop new and improved approaches for continuously improving the care of children with various chronic conditions.

6. Develop comprehensive pediatric case management/ care coordination, family education, and support programs through the managed care plan to enable both the primary and specialty physicians to more efficiently use their time and improve families' satisfaction with care.

7. Create ongoing education and training opportunities within the managed care plan for primary care physicians and specialists (including adult specialists serving children) in state-of-the-art approaches for the evaluation, diagnosis, and treatment of chronic childhood conditions.

8. Work with each family to help them understand how the managed care plan operates in terms of service coverage and authorization policies.

9. Work with the managed care plan to explore options to implement a health status adjustment to the capitation rate (ie, ACGs).

In closing, physician decision makers should not be controlled by the cost issue, but by medical judgment—capitated risk situations should not be structured to make the physician suffer financially for providing care to this vulnerable population.

## Contributing Authors

- Judith Palfrey, MD
- Marilynn Haynie, MD
- AAP Medical Home Program for Children With Special Needs

Reprinted from an insert in *AAP News*, February 1996.

# EFFECTIVE STRATEGIES FOR WORKING WITH MANAGED CARE PROGRAMS: AN ARIZONA PRACTICE SHARES ITS EXPERIENCES

## by Marcia Di Verde

The managed care movement of the early 1980s has become the emerging health issue of the 1990s.

There are some pediatricians who have avoided contracting with managed care health plans, being accustomed to and thriving financially with fee-for-service, but this may not be the case in the near future.

Two Arizona pediatricians have found that the adjustment to managed care has worked in their practice. David Hirsch, MD, FAAP, and Thomas Barela, MD, FAAP, of Phoenix, AZ, practice in a state whose entire special needs health care system is run by managed care health plans. Under these plans, all children in the state with special needs who qualify under Title XIX in the state are automatically enrolled in a managed care plan.

As many as 10% of the patients in the practice of Drs Hirsch and Barela are special needs children, many of whom are severely disabled. In 1989, the practice began contracting with managed care health plans for these children. Drs Hirsch and Barela, partners with Gerald H. Golner, and Pamela S. Murphy, MD, FAAP, at Phoenix Pediatrics, found that one of the most difficult aspects of caring for this population is coordinating referrals and follow-up from pediatric subspecialists.

"We learned within the first year of accepting these children in our practice that coordination with subspecialists and follow-up was a full-time job," said Dr Barela. "We've hired a care coordinator who now handles all of the referrals and follow-up. Following the procedures of the health plan is of the utmost importance. With the growing number of well-patients enrolled in managed care plans, all patients benefit from this specialized care coordination."

Drs Barela and Hirsch have placed themselves in an important negotiating position with the local health plan. Through analysis and careful tracking of patient data, they took to the bargaining table important statistics, vital in determining reimbursement rates for the children in their practice.

Reimbursement rates for well-children and children with special needs should be negotiated separately. "To do this you must know what it costs for their treatment," said Dr Barela. "Early in the process we reviewed old costs and set up a system for tracking current costs. We monitor all pharmaceutical dispensing, hospital, and office visits on an ongoing basis."

Subsequently, they found that the cost of physician services for children with special needs was more than twice the cost than for well-children. They also found more interesting data regarding care of children with special needs:

- Office visits were 1.5 times more frequent than those for well-children.

- Hospitalization rates were 5 to 10 times greater than those for well-children.

- Medical care required 2 to 3 times more physician time as that required for well-children, yet generated only 1.5 times as much income per office call.

While this discrepancy promotes pediatricians' reluctance to care for a large number of these children, this data can be an effective tool when negotiating with insurance and health plans.

Poor discharge planning is a common obstacle to providing continuity of care for children with special needs in a managed care plan. To avoid this, members of the group practice are on call and make hospital rounds for an entire week at a time. Since these children generally require longer and more frequent hospital stays, the physicians are able to provide patients and their families consistent health care coverage.

Another problem encountered when a practice accepts a significant number of patients with special needs is training. When the partners at Phoenix Pediatrics made the commitment to treat these children, they found that their formal pediatric education was lacking in out-patient care for special needs children.

"We had to train ourselves how to change G-tubes and tracheostomies in the office. The local OB-GYN practices were reluctant to do routine gynecologic exams for the special needs adolescent and young adult patients so we've developed the skill within our own practice," said Dr Barela.

"We've learned a lot about treating children with special needs in our practice, and we're continuing to do so," he added. "We are finding ways to improve or maintain quality of care for these children and looking for ways to reduce costs. We've been able to negotiate better rates with the health plan, not because we are skimping on care, but because we are becoming more efficient and effective in medical treatment for our patients."

If you would like more information about Phoenix Pediatrics' experiences with treating children with special needs under managed care, contact Drs Barela and Hirsch at 602/242-5121.

Reprinted from *CATCH Quaterly*, January 1995

# IMPROVING PRIMARY HEALTH SERVICES TO CHILDREN WITH CHRONIC ILLNESSES

## by W. Carl Cooley, MD, FAAP; Ardis L. Olson, MD, FAAP; and Jeanne McAllister, RN, MS

Children with chronic illnesses and disabilities can make up 20% of a primary care pediatric practice. Providing care to these children can be frustrating and challenging for pediatricians who are serving this vulnerable and complex population.

These frustrations generally fall into three categories: time, information, and coordination. First, quality primary care services for children with chronic conditions are time-consuming. As the managed care industry thrives, primary care physicians receive the same capitation rate for children with complicated problems as they do for other children. There is little financial incentive under most managed care plans to spend extra time on complex problems and some insurers discourage primary care providers from attracting children with high-cost health care needs into their practices.

Second, many primary care physicians feel inadequately informed about managing chronic illnesses and disabilities.

Finally, children with chronic illnesses often require extensive care coordination that involves the entire community. Communication between health care providers can run the gamut from fair to inadequate. Sometimes there is no coordination at all and in other cases children have multiple case managers who fail to communicate with one another.

In an effort to help primary care physicians reconcile these challenges, the Office Partners Project at the Dartmouth Hitchcock Medical Center in Lebanon, NH, has been working with 10 primary care pediatric practices in the state. Our aim is to assist each practice in the development of an effective and efficient Chronic Condition Management program (CCM). Pediatric practices can strengthen their services to children with special health care needs with a well-planned management approach that is part of the medical home model. The CCM program earmarks specific children for extra services in the primary care setting and improves the following:

- access to office services
- responsiveness to family needs
- care coordination
- office efficiency and reimbursement

## Lessons Learned

Several lessons have been learned through the Office Partners Project that will help pediatricians design a similar management program in their offices. In developing a CCM program, a group of parents of children with chronic conditions meet informally to provide the family perspective. Such input will help office staff determine what elements of the practice are helpful and what areas could be improved.

As parents are increasingly regarded as partners in their children's care, there are other ways practices can involve parents to improve care. Physicians should support parents in the development of expertise and provide confidence in advocating for their children's needs.

Another helpful model is connecting parents of children with similar conditions with other parents in the practice. For example, consider the creation of a parent advisory group to the practice. This group could have a bulletin board in the waiting area that provides information and materials for other parents. Another helpful tip is to give the parents a notebook to store their child's medical, social, and financial data.

## Adopt a Whole Office Systems Approach

Serving children with chronic conditions requires the involvement of the entire office. This means not only the participation of all personnel, but the examination of most aspects of office operations, including appointments, records, billing, and waiting room accommodations.

Before committing to a CCM program, office staff should meet and consider the comments of families of children with special needs. The office will probably be changing to become more responsive to these children and their families. Examples of specific interventions include the following:

- color-coded stickers on charts to identify children participating in the office's CCM program

- an office nurse designated as the practice's CCM facilitator

- a list for the receptionist showing which children are in the CCM program to ensure prompt attention and adequate time for the patient

## Communication Means Everything

Good care coordination must be an explicit process. Frequently, families, primary care physicians, and specialists have failed to communicate explicitly about their expectations concerning roles, responsibilities, and needs. Primary health care providers, however, are well positioned to break this cycle of incorrect expectations.

The primary care physician should communicate explicitly with specialists about the nature and scope of a consultation and the subsequent level of their anticipated involvement. The practice might consider developing a simple template for referrals to specialists or specialty clinics that would outline the concerns of the family and of the primary care physician and state to what degree on-going specialty care is desired.

Groups of pediatricians in community practice could request case-based continuing education programs on topics in Chronic Condition Management from a nearby tertiary care medical center or teaching hospital. This not only provides education but fosters better communication and coordination between primary and specialty care.

## Know Your Community's Resources

Pediatricians must be familiar with their state and local resources that may benefit children with special health care needs and their families. Some states provide family support services including respite care, service coordination, financial assistance, and advocacy to eligible children.

Most states have programs for children with special health care needs that provide a range of services from clinics and financial assistance to in-service training, parent-to-parent referral, and care coordination. Offices should develop community resource directories and identify an office staff person as the "house expert" about state and local resources for families.

Pediatricians need to review their billing practices for children with special health care needs carefully. In cases in which fee-for-service billing occurs, pediatricians may underestimate the time involved in specific patient encounters; this results in under-billing. Furthermore, services such as case management, counseling, and consultation with school or early intervention teams can be billable activities. Practices should discuss specific agreements with managed care providers to provide primary care services to specific children with extremely complex health care needs. Some managed care companies may be willing to negotiate primary care contracts to cover a broad range of reasonable primary care services for such children at higher capitation fees or to allow for fee-for-service billing.

### More about the program

Office Partners is a project of the Hood Center for Family Support in the Department of Pediatrics at the Dartmouth Hitchcock Medical Center in Lebanon, NH, and the New Hampshire University Affiliated Program. The project is supported through grant MCJ-337062-02 from the federal Maternal and Child Health Bureau and a grant from the Robert Wood Johnson Foundation. Office Partners is a component of an effort to develop comprehensive community-based services for children with special health care needs called New Hampshire Partners in Health. More information and a catalog of Chronic Condition Management materials is available by contacting the authors through Sandi Cragin at 603/650-8268, or by writing the Hood Center for Family Support, Dartmouth Hitchcock Medical Center, One Medical Center Drive, Lebanon, NH, 03756.

Reprinted from *CATCH Quarterly*, November 1995

# INDIANA PEDIATRICIAN WORKS TO COORDINATE SERVICES FOR CHILDREN WITH SPECIAL NEEDS

## by Marcia Di Verde

Rather than reinvent the wheel, John Poncher, MD, FAAP, of Valparaiso, IN, is using his CATCH planning funds to build on a successful venture that brings together leaders from health, education, and parent organizations. This group is charged with improving health services for children with special needs.

Since the group's formation in 1991, as many as 30 people have been attending the monthly meeting, which is referred to as the "Issues and Perspectives Group." The group's representatives are its secret weapon for its success. It includes members of the AAP Indiana Chapter, the Indiana Parent Information Network, State Board of Health, State Medicaid Department, Title V agency, Division of Special Education, and other organizations. Because the AAP Indiana Chapter feels a strong alliance with the group focusing on children with special needs, the 90-minute meetings dovetail with the AAP chapter's monthly gatherings.

These meetings have made a lasting impact on all parties. Now there is communication between agencies and organizations where there had previously been none. For instance, the group is tackling the issue of what is the best way to coordinate case management services among practitioners and state health agencies.

The Issues and Perspectives group has built a valuable rapport by working cooperatively with many organizations. They have been called upon to address reimbursement issues with the Medicaid agency; to enhance EPSDT Services; and to work with the state Division of Special Education to develop a video on how to manage medically fragile children in schools.

Julia Tipton Hogan, a policy analyst with the Indiana Medicaid Program, said the Issues and Perspectives group is the vehicle that brings all of the players together. She believes this forum will lead to a more comprehensive health system for children with complex medical needs.

The activity of the Issues and Perspectives Group is a classic example of CATCH at work. In this case, CATCH is bringing together state health and education officials and other organizations to help children. Many Indiana pediatricians feel connected to this program. Dr Poncher, who practices community pediatrics, said, "I have been a part of the group because there is a genuine commitment from all members to improve service delivery for children by working cooperatively."

The $10,000 CATCH planning funds, which are supported by Wyeth Pediatrics, have allowed Dr Poncher to hire consultant Joanne Martin, DrPH, MS, to help develop a medical home model for coordinating state agencies and providers that deliver services to children with special needs. The grant also enables Dr Martin to coordinate a retreat for the group to get their input on various matters. Dr Martin will also have the responsibility of writing a grant for funding to support the implementation of the group's activities.

For more information about the Medical Home Program for Children With Special Needs, please contact Liz Osterhus at 800/433-9016, ext 7621.

John Poncher, MD, is a partner with Associated Pediatricians in Valparaiso, IN. If you would like more information about the Issues and Perspectives Group, please contact Dr Poncher at 219/464-7460.

Reprinted from *CATCH Quarterly*, April 1995

# URBAN NATIVE AMERICAN CHILDREN WITH SPECIAL NEEDS OBTAIN NECESSARY SERVICES

## by Liz Osterhus

Native American families who have a child with special needs are often required to leave their homes on the reservation and move to the city so that their special needs child can get the necessary medical and social services. Once in the city, these Native Americans are removed from their extended family and the social support system available to them on their reservation. Due to cultural barriers and a lack of familiarity with the urban environment, these families have great difficulty coordinating the medical and nonmedical services they need on their own.

Several years ago, while bicycling on a hot, dry day in Albuquerque, NM, five pediatricians developed a plan to reduce the barriers to services for these families. Among the pedaling pediatricians was Lance Chilton, MD, chairperson of the American Academy of Pediatrics (AAP) Committee on Native American Child Health. The ideas that Dr Chilton and his colleagues generated that day became the foundation for the Helping Indian Children of Albuquerque (HICA) program.

The HICA program is a 5-year project funded in part by the federal Maternal and Child Health Bureau (MCHB) through a grant awarded under the Healthy Tomorrows Partnership for Children Program. The program's goal is to provide service coordination to Native American children who live in urban Albuquerque and have a suspected or diagnosed disability or chronic illness. The HICA staff help parents of urban Native American children with special needs identify community resources so that families can choose the most appropriate services for their child. The program staff visit the families at their homes, accompany them to medical appointments, attend school meetings, and provide any additional assistance the family may need to schedule and keep needed appointments.

Sandra Taft, a speech and hearing specialist with experience providing services to Native American families on reservations, was appointed the HICA

project director. Ms Taft ensures that the program is sensitive to both the cultural needs of urban Native American families and the practical needs of the pediatricians who provide services to these families. According to Ms Taft, the HICA program enables families to have "a voice." Without the program, "the families would be lost in the system" and important needs would not be met.

Prior to the HICA program, pediatricians caring for children with special needs and their families would have to single-handedly identify and refer these children to all the medical, social, educational, and financial services they require. This process was time-consuming, inefficient, and extremely difficult for pediatricians who manage a busy office practice.

The Service Coordinator of the HICA program, Catherine Riley, now acts as the care coordinator and ensures that all appointments are kept and all non-medical needs of the child and family are being met. Knowing that Ms Riley will attend to the nonmedical needs of the child and family allows the pediatrician to focus on medical issues and thereby be available to more families in need of services. "Without Cathy (the HICA service coordinator), we'd be overwhelmed," states Paul Dean Avritt, MD, one of the pediatricians involved in the HICA program.

In addition to the funding the program receives from the MCHB, the Levi Strauss Corporation has also provided funding to support the development of training materials for families and professional staff. The HICA program staff have already adapted a training program for Native American families with special needs children to teach parents how to be effective advocates for their children. The parents receive this training after they have been referred to needed services and have become active participants in the program.

The HICA program is an exemplary model of activities promoted and supported by the Medical

Home Program for Children With Special Needs (MHPCSN). The MHPCSN, a program housed in the AAP Department of Community Pediatrics, supports pediatricians who provide services to children with special needs. For more information about the MHPCSN, please contact Liz Osterhus at 800/433-9016, ext 7621.

Reprinted from *CATCH Quarterly*, Fall 1996

# Assuring Quality of Care for Children With Special Needs in Managed Care Organizations: Roles for Pediatricians

Henry T. Ireys, PhD; Holly A. Grason, MA; and Bernard Guyer, MD, MPH

**ABSTRACT.** Increasing numbers of children with special health care needs are enrolling in managed care programs. Although managed care may improve service coordination and use of primary care, it may also threaten health outcomes for these children by potentially decreasing access to the range of needed services, eroding progress in developing community-based service systems, and failing to assure quality of care. To date, few frameworks have been proposed to assess quality of care for this population of children in managed care organizations. In this article, we adapt the Institute of Medicine's definition of quality and identify six key components: content of service delivery systems, the nature of desired health outcomes, risks associated with service delivery, constraints of care, interpersonal dimensions, and attention to developmental issues. These components can be assessed at three levels: the individual, the health plan, and the community. Pediatricians and other child health professionals have critical roles to play in assuring that policies and practices within managed care organizations promote a high quality of care for this vulnerable population of children. *Pediatrics* 1996;98:178–185; *children with special needs, managed care, disabilities, chronic illness, quality of care.*

ABBREVIATIONS. SSI, Supplemental Security Income; CSHCN, Children With Special Health Care Needs; HMO, health maintenance organization; IOM, Institute of Medicine.

As states implement health system reforms, new problems are emerging in the organization and financing of care for children with disabilities and chronic illnesses. Many families, pediatricians, and other health care professionals are concerned that managed care programs in both the public and private sectors will decrease access to needed subspecialty and supportive services and undermine recent efforts to develop community-based systems of care for these children and their families.[1,2] Increased monitoring of medical costs and greater recognition of limited public resources will raise difficult questions about support for children who require long-term health and education services. Moreover, statewide implementation of Medicaid-managed care

From the Child and Adolescent Health Policy Center, Department of Maternal and Child Health, School of Hygiene and Public Health, Johns Hopkins University, Baltimore.
Received for publication Apr 4, 1995; accepted Sep 4, 1995.
Reprint requests to (H.T.I.) Department of Maternal and Child Health, 624 North Broadway, Baltimore, MD 21205.
PEDIATRICS (ISSN 0031 4005). Copyright © 1996 by the American Academy of Pediatrics.

programs and reductions in state Medicaid expenditures may affect this population disproportionately.

Little baseline data are available to assess the influence of these changes on health status and quality of life for these children and their families. As a result, pediatricians, other child health practitioners, families, and administrators of managed care programs will need to work together closely to balance cost-related concerns with assurances for a high quality of services for this population of children. Quality assessment for this population requires a broad strategy that encompasses physical health, mental health, social interaction, and family functioning. In this article, we aim to provide a framework for assessing quality of care for children with disabilities and chronic illnesses within the context of managed care programs and to identify key roles that pediatricians and other child health providers can play in assuring quality of care as health system reforms are implemented.

## OVERVIEW OF POPULATION CHARACTERISTICS AND COSTS OF CARE

In the adult population, there are a limited number of major chronic diseases and disabilities, including stroke-related conditions, cardiovascular disorders, cancer, and orthopedic conditions. Each of them, however, occurs with comparatively high frequency. In the child population, the pattern is reversed: more than 200 chronic conditions and disabilities affect youth, including asthma, diabetes, sickle cell anemia, spina bifida, epilepsy, and autism. With the exception of asthma, most of these conditions are rare.

Analyses of data from the 1988 National Health Interview Survey suggest that 31% of children less than 18 years of age (about 20 million children) have one or more chronic health conditions, excluding chronic mental health problems and learning disabilities.[3] Children with two or more chronic health conditions (2.2 million children) are at substantial risk for high rates of service use.[4] Many of the challenges faced by the families of these children are similar, regardless of the child's particular diagnosis.[5]

Children with disabilities and chronic illnesses represent the high-cost segment of the childhood population; although few in number, they consume a vastly disproportionate amount of service dollars. Issues of cost pertain directly to the scope of benefit packages developed by managed care organizations for children with special health care needs, to referral practices, and to adjustments made in the cost of premiums.

Detailed estimates of the costs of care are unavailable for this population as a whole. However, general estimates have been made for some subgroups. For example, incremental costs (ie, costs for services beyond what healthy children require) of medical care for children who have limitations in their activities are estimated to have exceeded $6.5 billion in 1992.[6] On average, a child with a disability cost Medicaid approximately $7100 in 1992, seven times more than a child with no disabilities.[7] Blackman[8] estimated that average hospital costs for the smallest surviving preterm infants exceeded $100 000 in 1990 and that hospital costs for a very low birth weight infant (less than 1000 g) were three to four times higher than costs for infants weighing more than 1500 g at birth. Average health expenditures for children with mental retardation were $4000 in the mid-1980s–four times the average expenditure for a healthy child.[9]

Studies also suggest that costs vary considerably within diagnostic categories. For example, a recent study found that incremental life-span economic costs for children with various heart defects ranged from $69 000 to $209 000.[10] In the mid-1980s, per capita annual health care expenditures in a national sample of youth with severe mental retardation were found to range from less than $100 to $43 000.[9] This variation typically results from the inclusion of a few children with extremely high medical care costs. Consequently, median expenditures are typically much lower than mean expenditures for most diagnostic groups within this population. Despite extensive within group variation in annual costs and mean expenditures, the majority of children with disabilities or chronic illnesses will not incur exorbitant medical expenditures within any given year. Predicting annual or lifetime costs for individual children in this population is difficult, however, because of the need to account for many demographic and health-related variables and the complex interactions among development, health status, and family environment.

## CHILDREN WITH SPECIAL NEEDS IN MANAGED CARE PROGRAMS

Managed care programs are quickly becoming the dominant organizational form in the health care system of the United States. Unfortunately, early studies of the effects of managed care on health outcomes of children are generally inconclusive and shed little light on the population of children with special needs.[11,12] The structural diversity and rapid development of these programs has far outpaced the knowledge needed to assess their impact on the health status of children with special health needs. Furthermore, the transition from a largely fee-for-service system to a managed care system poses special threats to existing relationships between families and health care practitioners. These relationships are often critical to effective management of the care of children.

To date, most managed care plans have not actively enrolled this population or developed special programs to address their needs. In the private sec-

tor, managed care plans have developed special patient education programs (eg, education around asthma management designed to reduce emergency department care or hospitalization). Overall, however, managed care programs have few incentives to extend coverage to children with disabilities or chronic illnesses. In the public sector, children with disabilities or chronic illnesses are usually exempted (or carved out) from many Medicaid-managed care plans.[13] In 1993, for example, 50% of the states that had mandatory enrollment of Medicaid clients into managed care programs exempted certain categories of children with special health care needs; more than 50% of the states that had voluntary enrollment in managed care plans excluded disabled Supplemental Security Income (SSI) recipients from participation.[2] Some states, such as Tennessee, have implemented mandatory managed care programs for the Medicaid-eligible population, yet have made no special provisions for children with disabilities or chronic conditions.[3]

In a few sites, special efforts have been made to develop managed care programs specifically for children with special needs.[14] Under the Section 1115 Medicaid managed care waiver in Kentucky, for example, children with special needs are assigned a case manager; special policies are being developed that will allow specialists and other providers to be the case managers and to maintain ongoing relationships with children currently under their care, assuming that these practitioners are willing to provide primary health care. In Michigan, the state Title V program for Children With Special Health Care Needs (CSHCN) has developed a physician case management model for this group of children in managed care programs.[15] One of the major challenges is to understand the implications of structural variations that are emerging in managed care programs.[16] A further challenge for managed care programs (and the field generally) involves defining the boundaries for this population. Definitional approaches have been discussed at length,[17,18] but a standard approach has yet to be widely adopted by managed care organizations. This lack of a standard definition is inhibiting the development of managed care service delivery models for this population.

## CRITICAL AREAS OF CONCERN

The adequacy of the current health service system for children with disabilities and chronic illnesses has been debated at length.[5] From our perspective, major concerns tend to cluster around seven key issues: 1) access to care; 2) appropriateness of services; 3) comprehensiveness; 4) coordination; 5) continuity; 6) relation to community; and 7) the degree to which services and the service system are family-centered. All seven issues are relevant to the traditional indemnity insurance system. The increased inclusion of this population into managed care systems may exacerbate certain problems (eg, access to care), but also may bring new opportunities to address other longstanding problems in the current service system (eg, continuity of care). To make our discussion manageable, we focus on three cross-cutting areas: access to services, gaps in the service system, and quality of care.

*Access to services.* Numerous concerns have been raised regarding reduced access to pediatric subspecialists in managed care programs, thereby leading to failures in detecting emerging problems, delays in using new medications or treatments, or applications of inappropriate treatments. Fox and colleagues report that benefit packages offered by health maintenance organizations (HMOs) that contract with state Medicaid programs are less comprehensive than packages provided under the standard Medicaid fee-for-service plans.[19] A study of Aid to Families With Dependent Children recipients receiving Medicaid services in Wisconsin indicated that fewer than 50% of respondents who had requested a referral to an out-of-plan specialist were granted one.[20] Reporting on a survey of administrators of 22 managed care plans, Fox and McManus[6] noted that with some exceptions, "few plans have made special efforts to assure the appropriate participation of pediatric specialists in their provider networks. This fact . . . often makes it difficult for families whose children have special health care needs to access appropriate pediatric specialists."

A study of barriers to pediatric referral found that managed care systems are successful in restricting referrals to pediatric subspecialists and to inpatient care. Pediatricians with patients covered under managed care and fee-for-service systems report making fewer referrals to subspecialists and to inpatient care for patients in managed care programs compared with those in fee-for-service programs.[21] In the group of pediatricians who had made referrals to pediatric subspecialists for patients in managed care programs, one fifth indicated that at least one referral was denied; of those reporting at least one denial, about one third said they believed that the patient's health was compromised as a result of the denial.[1]

Access to health-related services (eg, physical therapy) also may be limited by managed care programs through policies that restrict duration of services, limit total number of encounters, or establish special conditions under which services can be provided.[6]

Some studies suggest that managed care programs increase access to and use of primary care services and decrease use of emergency departments for non-Medicaid children in comparison to fee-for-service arrangements.[23,24] Few investigations of this topic have controlled for children with special needs. However, a recent study of 1685 children receiving Medicaid who were randomly assigned to fee-for-service or HMO programs did account for the presence of major disabling conditions (blindness, diabetes, cerebral palsy, mental retardation, and amputations) and allergies (eczema, asthma, and hay fever). The investigators report that children with these conditions in the HMO had as many check-up and acute care visits as did children with these conditions in the fee-for-service system,[25] suggesting few differences in use of health services. Several factors, however, limit generalizability of these results: data were collected over a 2-month period, the number of

children with major disabling conditions was small, and only one HMO was studied.

*Gaps in the service system.* In theory, managed care systems will promote access to comprehensive primary care as a strategy to detect problems early and prevent secondary health conditions and may enhance service coordination by virtue of gatekeeping procedures. However, primary care physicians now vary widely in the nature and extent of their experience in providing services to children with special needs,[26,27] and may be unfamiliar with new or emerging treatment protocols for children with particular diagnoses. Under some types of managed care programs, subspecialists may serve as gatekeepers and will manage their patients' primary care needs. How these different arrangements affect health outcomes is unknown.

Children with special health care needs are dependent on a wide range of community institutions to receive needed educational, social, recreational, and vocational services. Orchestrating the relevant agencies and programs into a coherent and nonduplicative set of services is essential for effective health care, but it also requires continuing effort in the face of ongoing changes in program staff, eligibility criteria, and enrollment procedures. To coordinate services, pediatricians and other child health providers must interact with numerous state and federal programs, including the Title V programs for CSHCN, local programs under the Individuals with Disabilities Education Act, the SSI program, and Head Start. Managed care organizations may have little experience or incentive to establish necessary linkages with these programs at the community level.

It is noteworthy also that in many states, education agencies bill Medicaid for health-related services rendered by school personnel to Medicaid-enrolled students in special education programs. As Medicaid includes more children with special needs in managed care programs, many issues will be raised concerning payment for these services. Available data suggest that managed care organizations have yet to incorporate provisions for negotiating financial and referral arrangements with special education programs.[28]

*Assessing quality.* The growth in managed care programs has been accompanied by concerns that attention to limiting costs also will limit quality of services for children with disabilities and chronic illnesses.[29] In particular, few state Medicaid agencies have incorporated safeguards pertaining to these children into their contracts with managed care organizations. Although some efforts have been made to develop pertinent standards and quality indicators for this population of children,[30] little attention has been paid to conceptualizing quality as it relates to this population. Because issues of quality are critical to both pediatricians involved in the care of these children and administrators of managed care organizations, it is worth considering in depth how quality can be conceptualized for this population.

## CONCEPTS OF QUALITY

The Institute of Medicine (IOM) defines quality of care as "the degree to which health services for individuals and populations increase the likelihood of desired health outcomes and are consistent with current professional knowledge."[31] Harris-Wehling[32] provides a useful review of the components underlying this definition. Somewhat adapted and expanded, these components provide a conceptual framework for assessing quality of care for children with special needs and their families.

*Content of care.* The term **health services** was deliberately included in the IOM's definition of quality of care because it refers to a wide range of elements of care, extending beyond more narrow terms such as **medical services**. This approach is especially relevant for children with special needs. A narrow focus on subspecialty medical care ignores other essential services such as primary care, developmentally appropriate assistive technology, or community-based family support programs. These services can have important direct and indirect effects on health status by influencing quality of family life, adherence to medical treatments, and capacity to cope with stresses commonly associated with childhood disability or chronic illness. The outcome of even the most brilliant surgical procedure to correct an infant's birth defect can be undermined by inadequate resources for the family to provide postsurgical care at home. This fact requires us to take a broader perspective on the essential components of care for these children and their families.

*Goals of care.* What are **desired health outcomes**? Pediatricians, parents, and children themselves may answer these questions differently. For health care practitioners, answers often involve measurable technical or biomedical achievements (eg, increasing range of motion in a particular limb). For parents, treatment goals may be developmental in nature (eg, not restricting an active child with orthopedic interventions or invasive treatments). For the youth themselves, goals may involve quality-of-life issues that are inconsistent with certain medical interventions. Moreover, different goals may be relevant depending on whether the child is in the hospital or at home. Trade-offs between costs of providing care and potential benefits almost always shape the process of setting treatment goals. These potential complexities in defining **desirable** health outcomes imply that quality of care is inherently relativistic and relational; assessments of quality depend on the person making the judgment, the relationship between that person and the child, and the setting in which judgments are made.

*Risk of care.* Outcomes of health services can not be guaranteed because every health service has some risk for poor or unintended outcomes. The IOM's definition of quality of care accounts for this observation by noting that health services can only increase the **likelihood** of desired outcomes. This concept is especially pertinent to this population of children because new medical treatments for this population emerge routinely. Long-term risks of some treatments may not be completely known before widespread adoption. Knowledge of risk and benefit ratios may alter the availability of financing, which in turn may shape the diffusion of treatment innovations for this group of children. One dimension of assessing quality within managed care programs must involve questions of how new treatments are diffused into standard benefit packages as well as the broader question of how treatment decisions balance estimates of risk and benefit within an environment highly conscious of cost implications.

*Constraints on care.* The IOM definition explicitly recognizes that quality of care is limited by **current professional knowledge**. The effectiveness of many technologies and procedures is not known, and this is especially true for many services related to the population of children with disabilities and chronic illnesses. Medical protocols vary from clinic to clinic, with little comparative evidence to favor one method over another. Variance is especially extreme with respect to generally accepted standards for providing family support services, in part because knowledge about their effectiveness is sparse. It is difficult to judge quality of a procedure if the underlying research base on its effectiveness is absent or inconclusive. Moreover, if a treatment has not been shown to be efficacious, then it is less likely to be considered medically necessary. Knowledge about effectiveness of medical procedures shapes definitions of **medical necessity**, which in turn influence availability of insurance coverage.[33]

Other types of constraints can be placed on care as well, including financial constraints. For example, some services may be technically feasible but financially exorbitant, either to society or to the family. In fact, many families have had to confront the difficult questions of paying for expensive care or modifications to the home at the expense of resources for other family members. To what extent should providers and health care institutions account for these economic constraints in assessing quality of care? This issue also arises when providers and families differ regarding judgments in the overuse of certain technologies. For example, repetition of expensive lab tests that involve invasive procedures may be perceived as important by providers but financially burdensome by families or health plan administrators.

*Interpersonal dimensions of care.* Many definitions of quality stress both the technical competence of providers and the interpersonal **art** of applying technical skills in the context of human relationships. No amount of interpersonal skill should overshadow technical shoddiness, nor should lack of interpersonal skill undermine technical brilliance. For most health care providers, competencies are needed in both the technical and interpersonal aspects of care. This is particularly true for health care professionals who will be involved with families over a long period of time.

Harris-Wehling[32] extends this notion further by invoking the concept of a practitioner's "fidelity to a community of patients." This concept suggests that pediatricians have an obligation to be technically proficient, interpersonally skilled, and committed to integrating family-centered practices and policies that will foster the health of all patients and families.[34,35] Especially important are skills related to the inclusion of families in decision-making and in managing the issues of informed choice when treatment goals are established. Issues of choice are particularly germane to professionals in managed care settings, when fidelity to the institution may conflict with the need to share information with families in an unbiased manner and to discuss the broadest range of choices possible.

*Developmental perspective.* For most children with chronic illnesses or disabilities, development and health status interact in a complex fashion. For example, a wheelchair that is suitable for a 5-year-old can become ill-fitting before age 6; for adolescents with physical disabilities, normative developmental anxieties around body image may contribute to serious secondary conditions such as eating disorders or depression. Moreover, as children progress through childhood to adolescence, it is expected that they will take increasing responsibility for self-care such as administering their own medication, reporting changes in symptoms, and interacting more directly with health professionals. To assist this process, health professionals need sufficient training in the application of developmental concepts to children and youth with chronic health problems. During the last two decades greater focus has been directed to conceptualizing and understanding how children actively use their own dispositional strengths and interpersonal skills to achieve positive developmental outcomes. Renewed concerns with concepts such as effectance motivation,[36] social competence,[37,38] and resilience[39] have begun to correct a disproportionate attraction to deficit-related concepts. This perspective emphasizes that many individuals with disabilities have considerable strengths and that an important goal of the health care system should be the promotion of competencies and prevention of secondary conditions. A focus on health promotion is consistent with the premise of managed care, but the development of effective health promotion efforts for children with special needs may require new strategies and programs particularly suited to this population.

## ROLES FOR PEDIATRICIANS

Over the last two decades, ambulatory care pediatricians and other primary care professionals have been encouraged to play active roles in the care of children with chronic health conditions by assisting families in managing the child's condition, by coordinating medical and health services, and by becoming a trusted source of guidance and advice for the family.[26,27,40] Most of these recommendations are based on the belief that by playing such active roles, pediatricians can improve the child's medical outcomes, avoid unnecessary interventions, and support the family in its role as primary caregiver. In many instances, however, the actual capacity of pe-

diatricians to play these roles is limited by constraints on time, the lack of reimbursement for these activities, and limited training.[40] These limitations may persist in an environment dominated by managed care organizations. However, managed care organizations also have the opportunities to provide a **medical home** for these children while continuing to monitor costs. The infrastructure of many large managed care organizations has the potential to support programs of comprehensive care that will increase satisfaction and improve outcomes of care. Furthermore, some managed care organizations have advanced information systems; the potential for these systems to assist in measuring and tracking quality of care in relation to outcomes is largely untapped. The challenge for pediatricians and other child health professionals is to work with the leadership of managed care organizations to assist in developing resource-constrained but appropriate service models[41] and to explore how information can be collected and used to improve quality of care.

Assessments of quality must extend beyond the level of the individual encounter between patient and practitioner to include also the health plan and the community-based system of care.[42] The six components of quality noted previously can be mapped against these three levels (individual, health plan, community) to suggest key activities that pediatricians and other child health practitioners can undertake in the process of assuring quality of care for these children.

**The Individual Level**

At the individual level, these six components reflect the elements of good patient care. The importance of attending to a wide range of needs, negotiating clear treatment goals with the family, acknowledging levels of risk and constraints of knowledge, and incorporating good interpersonal skills within a family-centered and developmental framework are tasks usually associated with high quality clinical care for this population of children. In addition, many families of children with special health care needs (even those who are already in capitated systems) are unfamiliar with the general concept of managed care or the specific implications of any single program. When questions arise, these families will turn to pediatricians who have provided medical care, guidance, and support. Thus, pediatricians also will need to play critical roles in educating families regarding new choices and challenges, and assisting them in negotiating the transition to managed care.

Quality of care at the individual level will also depend on how successfully individual pediatricians in managed care organizations balance the ethical conflicts inherent in the gatekeeping role. Primary care pediatricians may feel pressure to **stretch their competence** and not refer patients to specialists to conserve either their own or an organization's resources. This practice conflicts with their primary obligation to serve the needs of their patients.[43] Although some **bedside rationing** is inevitable in any health care financing system, managed care organizations have an obligation to develop fair practice guidelines for primary care pediatricians and other health professionals to assure that children who require specialty care are not placed at a disadvantage. Pediatricians need to be actively involved in the development of such guidelines.[40]

## The Health Plan Level

Strategies for assuring quality of care at the health plan level involve some activities that are familiar to most pediatricians. Other tasks, however, may lead pediatricians into new territory. Table 1 lists potential tasks associated with the six components of quality at the health plan level. It illustrates, for example, the need to define an appropriately broad benefit package as a means for defining the content of care within health plans for this population of children. Furthermore, pediatricians and other child health professionals can play important roles in assisting administrators in managed care organizations to develop measures or indices of satisfaction and developmental appropriateness. One large managed care organization completed over 50 000 satisfaction surveys in 1994; few, however, were focused on this population.[44] Pediatricians, families, and research staff in managed care organizations will need to work together to develop satisfaction surveys that will contribute to family-centered policies and practices.[4,3,45] Furthermore, as professionals who are knowledgeable about the interactions between development and health status, pediatricians will be responsible for examining the developmental implications of the policies and procedures of managed care programs.

For other components, many pediatricians and child health professionals will face concepts that have not been part of traditional service delivery systems. For example, much like the corporate sector's concern with new product development, managed care organizations place considerable emphasis on defining the value of an intervention, where value is viewed as the cost of a service balanced against its health benefits. From this perspective, costly interventions may be supported if they are known to have substantial benefits. Even inexpensive interventions, however, may be excluded from coverage unless there is evidence of their positive impact on health status. Defining the value of an intervention intersects with the task of defining the goals of care and therefore requires a careful integration of the diverse perspectives of the child, family, physician, and plan administrator. Some services may be of considerable value to families but have not been shown to have cost benefits to the plan. "Value to whom?" will be a

difficult question to resolve and the answer may be found only through a combination of expert judgment and family participation.

Related to the concept of defining an intervention's value is the concept of defining risk. Most managed care organizations are **risk-aversive**, meaning that interventions whose outcomes are uncertain will be less likely to be covered in a benefit package. Yet, parents of many children with chronic illnesses or disabilities are willing to take risks on new treatments even if there is only a small possibility for positive outcomes. How will these opposing perspectives be resolved? At what point will new technologies be integrated into benefit packages offered by a managed care organization? How will current knowledge about the rapidly-changing treatment picture for many chronic illnesses and disabilities be made available to the decision-makers in managed care organizations? Pediatricians will necessarily be key participants in decision-making around these matters.

The issue of adoption of new treatments is an example of the larger task of identifying the boundaries of professional knowledge. Health status varies widely across children with the same chronic illness or disability, reflecting differences in both the phenotypic expression of the disease process and the child's family and socioeconomic environment. At this point in time, knowledge is insufficient to define a rigid treatment protocol for all children with a given chronic condition. For the foreseeable future, clinical judgment will play an extremely important role in establishing treatment protocols for individual children. At the level of the health plan, how much room will be made for the role of clinical judgment? Too narrow a role (ie, standard protocols that fail to account for individual differences) will yield a poor quality of care; too wide a role may conflict with the goal of cost containment. Where is the right balance and how is this to be determined and monitored? Answers to these questions will require considerable input by a broad range of pediatricians and other child health professionals.

## The Community Level

At the community level, attention to these six components of quality involves core public health principles of needs assessment, monitoring of health status, and assurances of quality of care. Numerous strategies are available to accomplish these goals. For example, periodic population-based surveys can assess access to an appropriate set of services and satisfaction with the interpersonal and developmental dimensions of services received. Public health

**TABLE.** Components of Quality and Associated Activities at the Health Plan Level

| Components | Activities |
|---|---|
| Content | Identifying an appropriate benefits package |
| Interpersonal dimensions | Addressing family/child satisfaction with policies and procedures |
| Growth and development | Examining developmental implications of policies and procedures |
| Goals | Defining the value of interventions |
| Risk | Predicting outcomes and consequences of new treatments |
| Constraints | Determining the role of clinical judgment |

agencies, such as state programs for CSHCN, can play active roles in disseminating information about managed care organizations in general and results of performance reviews of specific managed care plans. These agencies also can serve to advance the knowledge of new treatments and the value of interventions by hosting consensus-building conferences and by developing and disseminating standards of care and best practice manuals. Some state agencies have begun to implement projects related to these goals (M. McPherson, personal communication).

To promote quality of care for the population of children with special needs in managed care programs, both internal and external reviews will be needed.[46] Managed care programs (as well as fee-for-service programs) must continue to conduct internal audits of service quality through a variety of review procedures, performance measures, and consumer satisfaction surveys. Established managed care organizations that have a large enrollment and substantial experience may have the resources to conduct these reviews successfully. But even careful audits by the large managed care organizations may not address: 1) those children who lack insurance altogether; 2) children who are enrolled in smaller health plans that lack adequate resources for assessing or assuring quality of care; 3) the special circumstances and needs of Medicaid-enrolled children with chronic illnesses and disabilities who may require special services (eg, transportation to service sites) that managed care programs have little experience in providing;[14] and 4) services (eg, day care for children with special needs) that lay outside of traditional medical treatments but which are essential components to a comprehensive community-based service system. Pediatricians will need to play an active role in seeking ways of assuring that these services are accessible and of assuring quality of care for disenfranchised or at-risk subgroups within this population.

One strategy for pediatricians involves participating in local interagency coordination councils established under PL 99–457 (Part H of the Individuals with Disabilities Education Act that mandates early intervention for infants or toddlers with or at risk for disabilities) or becoming knowledgeable about and serving as advisors to state programs for CSHCN, many of which have a long history of involving pediatricians in policy-setting and implementation.[47] For example, in some states, directors of state CSHCN programs have begun to assume active leadership by working with families to define models of managed care and schedules for rate-setting that are appropriate to this population.[6,48]

Far more effort will be needed as the diversity of managed care organizations increases and as diverse health system reforms are implemented among the states. Although many state CSHCN programs have met difficult challenges in linking with managed care organizations,[14] these state programs have played leadership roles in implementing reforms in previous decades and many programs have considerable experience in managing contracts with specialty providers. As a result, many of the state CSHCN programs are likely to become the primary vehicle for assuring quality of care for this population at the community level. Their success will depend heavily on partnerships with both specialty and general pediatricians.

## CONCLUSIONS

Pediatricians, including those within and outside of the public health system, have played and will continue to play an important role in assessing services for children with special health care needs and their families, assuring access to an appropriately broad range of services of high quality, and developing tools and strategies for promoting quality of care. Reforms in the structure and financing of health care are unlikely to diminish the importance of these roles. The specific activities associated with each of these roles, however, will need to evolve in response to the implementation of reforms. Selected communities and projects have demonstrated that effective, coordinated service systems for children with special needs can be developed using a family-centered framework based on developmental concepts, functional considerations, and the promotion of competencies.[45,49] With sustained advocacy and practical assistance from families, pediatricians, and other health providers, this progress will continue as health system reforms are implemented.

The current challenges are: 1) to assure that expansion of managed care programs does not erode the important achievements already accomplished and 2) to assist managed care programs in meeting the goal of providing a set of comprehensive services of high quality in the context of cost containment. Some of the key issues that must be resolved include: 1) using incentives to assure that quality of care, broadly defined, will be given sufficient attention within managed care programs and in a fashion that will promote fidelity to a community of these children and families, 2) resolving technical, measurement problems in relation to assessment of quality at various levels, and 3) revising or expanding the concept of **medical necessity** to account for the wide range of services needed by this population of children.

## ACKNOWLEDGMENTS

Preparation of this article was supported in part with National Academy of Sciences program initiation funds and by a Cooperative Agreement (MCU 243A19) from the Maternal and Child Health Bureau, Health Resources and Services Administration, Department of Health and Human Services.

This article is a revised version of a paper prepared for a workshop entitled "Strategies for Assuring the Provision of Quality Services Through Managed Care Delivery Systems to Children With Special Health Care Needs" held in December 1994 under the auspices of the Institute of Medicine with support from the Division of Services to Children With Special Health Care Needs, Maternal and Child Health Bureau, Health Resources and Services Administration, Department of Health and Human Services.

We are much indebted to Ms Jo Harris-Wehling, who provided considerable assistance and feedback during the preparation of the original manuscript and who orchestrated the Institute of Medicine's workshop, to Dr Merle McPherson for her continuing leadership and guidance, to Dr David Heppel for ongoing support of the Child and Adolescent Health Policy Center, and to Ms Lori

Friedenberg for considerable assistance in preparing the manuscript.

# REFERENCES

1. Institute of Medicine. *Strategies for Assuring the Provision of Quality Services Through Managed Care Delivery Systems to Children with Special Health Care Needs: Workshop Highlights.* Washington, DC: National Academy of Sciences; 1995

2. Fox HB, Wicks LB, Newacheck PW. State Medicaid health maintenance organization policies and special-needs children. *Health Care Financ Rev.* 1993;15:25–37

3. Newacheck PW, Taylor WR. Childhood chronic illness: prevalence, severity, and impact. *Am J Public Health.* 1992;82:364–371

4. Newacheck PW, Stoddard JJ. Prevalence and impact of multiple childhood chronic illnesses. *J Pediatr.* 1994;124:40–48

5. Hobbs N, Perrin J, Ireys H. *Chronically Ill Children and Their Families.* San Francisco, CA: Jossey-Bass; 1985

6. Newacheck PW, Hughes DC, McManus MM, Perrin JM, Valdez RB, Fox HB. *Meeting Children's Long Term Care Needs Under the Health Security Act's Home and Community-Based Services Program.* San Francisco, CA: Institute for Health Policy Studies, University of California at San Francisco; 1994

7. Regenstein M, Meyer JA. *Low Income Children with Disabilities: How Will They Fare Under Health Care Reform?* Portland, ME: National Academy for State Health Policy; 1994

8. Blackman JA, Healy A, Ruppert ES. Participation by pediatricians in early intervention: impetus from Public Law 99–457. *Pediatrics.* 1992;89:98–102

9. Birenbaum A, Guyot D, Cohen H. *Health Care Financing for Severe Developmental Disabilities.* In: Begab M, series editor. Monographs of the American Association on Mental Retardation, Number 14. Washington, DC: American Association on Mental Retardation; 1990

10. Waitzman NJ, Romano PS, Scheffler RM. Estimates of the economic costs of birth defects. *Inquiry.* 1994;31:188–205

11. Fox HB, McManus MA. *Medicaid Managed Care Arrangements and Their Impact on Children and Adolescents: A Briefing Report.* Washington, DC: Fox Health Policy Consultants; 1992

12. Valdez RB, Ware JE Jr, Manning WG, et al. Prepaid group practice effects on the utilization of medical services and health outcomes for children: results from a controlled trial [published erratum appears in *Pediatrics.* 1989;83:678]. *Pediatrics.* 1989;83:168–180

13. National Association of Children's Hospitals and Related Institutions. *Summary of Key Characteristics of Session 1115 Medicaid Managed Care Waivers.* Alexandria, VA: NACHRI; 1994

14. Fox HB, Nadesh P, McManus MA, Wicks LB. *A Preliminary Examination of State Medicaid Demonstration Waiver Programs and Children with Special Health Care Needs.* Washington, DC: Maternal and Child Health Policy Research Center; 1994

15. Subcommittee on the Managed Care Initiative. *Managed Care for Children with Special Health Care Needs: Physician Case Management Model.* Lansing, MI: Children's Special Health Care Services Program, Michigan Department of Public Health; 1995

16. Fox HB, McManus MA. *Preliminary Analysis of Issues and Options in Serving Children with Chronic Conditions Through Medicaid Managed Care Plans.* Portland, ME: National Academy for State Health Policy; 1994

17. Stein R, Coupey S, Bauman L, Westbrook L, Ireys H. Framework for identifying children who have chronic conditions: the case for a new definition. *J Pediatr.* 1993;122:342–347

18. Perrin E, Newacheck P, Pless IB, et al. Issues involved in the definition and classification of chronic health conditions. *Pediatrics.* 1993;91:787–793

19. Fox HB, Wicks LB, Newacheck PW. Health maintenance organizations and children with special health needs: a suitable match? *Am J Dis Child.* 1993;147:546–552

20. Brazner K, Gaylord G. *Medicaid, HMOs, and Maternal and Child Health: An Assessment of Wisconsin's Mandatory Enrollment Program for AFDC Families.* Madison, WI: Center for Public Representation; 1986

21. Cartland JD, Yudkowsky BK. Barriers to pediatric referral in managed care systems. *Pediatrics.* 1992;89:183–192

22. Horwitz SM, Stein RE. Health maintenance organizations vs indemnity insurance for children with chronic illness: trading gaps in coverage. *Am J Dis Child.* 1990;144:581–586

23. Manning WG, Leibowitz A, Goldberg GA, Rogers WH, Newhouse JP. A controlled trial of the effect of a prepaid group practice on use of services *N Engl J Med.* 1984;310:1505–1510

24. Perkoff GT, Kahn L, Haas PJ. The effects of an experimental prepaid group practice on medical care utilization and cost. *Med Care.* 1976;14:432–449

25. Mauldon J, Leibowitz A, Buchanan JL, Damberg C, McGuigan KA. Rationing or rationalizing children's medical care: comparison of a Medicaid HMO with fee-for-service care. *Am J Public Health.* 1994;84:899–904

26. Blancquaert IR, Zvagulis I, Gray-Donald K, Pless IB. Referral patterns for children with chronic diseases. *Pediatrics.* 1992;90:71–74

27. Young PC, Shyr Y, Schork MA. The role of the primary care physician in the care of children with serious heart disease. *Pediatrics.* 1994;94:284–290

28. Rivera L, Regan C, Rosenbaum S. *Managed Care and Children's Health: An Analysis of Early and Periodic Screening, Diagnosis, and Treatment Services Under State Medicaid Managed Care Contracts.* Los Angeles, CA: National Health Law Project; 1995

29. Newacheck PW, Hughes DC, Stoddard JJ, Halfon N. Children with chronic illness and Medicaid managed care. *Pediatrics.* 1994;93:497–500

30. Epstein SG, Taylor AB, Halberg AS, Gardner JD, Walker DK, Crocker AC. *Enhancing Quality. Standards and Indicators of Quality Care for Children with Special Health Care Needs.* Boston, MA: New England SERVE; 1989

31. Institute of Medicine. *Medicare: A Strategy for Quality Assurance, Volume I.* Washington, DC: National Academy Press; 1990

32. Harris-Wehling J. Defining quality of care. In: Lohr KN, ed. *Medicare: A Strategy for Quality Assurance: Volume II: Sources and Methods.* Washington, DC: National Academy Press; 1990

33. Jameson EJ, Wehr E. Drafting national health care reform legislation to protect the health interests of children. *Stanford Law & Policy Review.* 1993;Fall:152–176

34. Harrison H. The principles for family-centered neonatal care. *Pediatrics.* 1993;92:643–650

35. Hutchins VL, McPherson M. National agenda for children with special health needs: social policy for the 1990s through the 21st century. *Am Psychol.* 1991;46:141–143

36. White RW. Motivation reconsidered: the concept of competence. *Psychol Rev.* 1959;66:297–333

37. King GA, Shultz IZ, Steel K, Gilpin M, Cathers T. Self-evaluation and self-concept of adolescents with physical disabilities. *Am J of Occup Ther.* 1993;47:132–140

38. Zigler E, Trickett PK. IQ, social competence, and evaluation of early childhood intervention programs. *Am Psychol.* 1978;33:789–798

39. Garmezy N. Resilience in children's adaptation to negative life events and stressed environments. *Pediatr Ann.* 1991;20:459–466

40. Liptak GS, Revell GM. Community physician's role in case management of children with chronic illnesses. *Pediatrics.* 1989;84:465–471

41. Committee on Child Health Financing. Guiding principles for managed care arrangements for the health care of infants, children, adolescents, and young adults. *Pediatrics.* 1995;95:613–615

42. Durch JS, ed. *Protecting and Improving Quality of Care for Children Under Health Care Reform: Workshop Highlights.* Washington, DC: Institute of Medicine; 1994

43. Council on Ethical and Judicial Affairs, American Medical Association. Ethical issues in managed care. *JAMA.* 1995;273:330–335

44. Peterson E. *The Managed Care Provider Assuring Quality.* Presentation at the Children with Special Health Care Needs Continuing Education Seminar. Columbus, OH: Children's Hospital; 1995

45. Shelton TL, Stepanek JS. *Family-Centered Care for Children Needing Specialized Health and Developmental Services.* Bethesda, MD: Association for the Care of Children's Health; 1994

46. Lohr KN, Grossman JH, Cassel CK. Issues in measuring and assuring quality of care for health care reform. *JAMA.* 1993;270:1911

47. Ireys HT, Nelson R. New federal policy for children with special health care needs: implications for pediatricians. *Pediatrics.* 1992;90:321–327

48. Morris B, McCandless D. *A Study of the Feasibility of a Capitated Rate Setting System for the Children's Special Health Care Services (CSHCS) Program.* Lansing, MI: CSHCS Program, Michigan Department of Public Health; 1994

49. Bronheim SM, Keefe ML, Morgan CC. *Communities Can: Building Blocks of a Community Based System of Care.* Washington, DC: Georgetown University Child Development Center; 1993

# Capitation Adjustment for Pediatric Populations

Elizabeth J. Fowler, PhD* and Gerard F. Anderson, PhD‡

**ABSTRACT.** *Objective.* The objective of this study is to assess the predictive performance of current claims-based capitation adjustment methods for pediatric populations. Medicaid programs and other insurers may increasingly use these systems for capitation rate setting, physician profiling, and other purposes.

*Methods.* Five leading models, a demographic model, ambulatory care groups, ambulatory diagnostic groups, diagnostic cost groups, and payment amounts for capitated systems, were tested by using use and expenditure data for children enrolled in the Maryland Medicaid program and a private nonprofit health maintenance organization in Minnesota. The models were tested at the individual level by using multiple regression methods and at the group level by using split-half validation to create both random and nonrandom groups. One of the nonrandom groups was created to represent children with chronic conditions.

*Results.* The findings indicate that although each of the alternative methods offers an improvement over a demographic model, significant underpayment remained for high-risk children, regardless of the capitation adjustment method used.

*Conclusions.* It is concluded that children with chronic conditions would probably remain at risk for discrimination in a competitive health care market under all models tested. Limitations associated with current alternatives suggest the need for further research in the area of pediatric capitation adjustment methods. *Pediatrics* 1996;98:10–17; *managed care, health maintenance organization, rate setting, capitation, risk adjustment, Medicaid, chronic disease.*

ABBREVIATIONS. DCG, diagnostic cost group; PACS, payment amounts for capitated systems; ACG, ambulatory care group; ADG, ambulatory diagnostic group; MDC, major diagnostic category; ICD-9, International Classification of Diseases, ninth revision.

This study is intended to assess the predictive performance of current claims-based capitation adjustment methods for pediatric populations. These methods can be used to adjust capitation payment rates for health status to equalize the expected cost of treating healthy and sick enrollees. They are impor-

From the Institute for Research and Education, HealthSystem Minnesota, Minneapolis; and ‡Department of Health Policy and Management, Johns Hopkins University School of Hygiene and Public Health, Baltimore.

Preliminary results from this study were presented at the 12th Annual Meeting of the Association for Health Services Research, June 5, 1995, Chicago, IL.

Received for publication Aug 17, 1995; accepted Oct 6, 1995.

Reprint requests to (E.J.F.) Institute for Research and Education, HealthSystem Minnesota, 5000 W 39th St, Minneapolis, MN 55416.

tant because Medicaid programs and other insurers may increasingly use these systems for capitation rate setting, physician profiling, and other purposes.

Capitation payment rates can be used to pay managed care plans and providers on a prospectively determined per capita basis and is thought to promote efficiency in the health care system. One drawback, however, is that if the rate-setting method is such that a plan or provider is paid the same rate for a patient with chronic health problems as for a patient who is generally healthy, there is a financial incentive to avoid enrolling patients with more serious illnesses.[1,2] This is known as selection bias.

Deliberate action on the part of managed care plans to enroll a population with better health risks is called "cream skimming," and the resulting low-risk population is referred to as favorable selection. Health plans can achieve a patient population of better health risks by enrolling healthier individuals, by discouraging enrollment by high-risk individuals, or by encouraging high-risk individuals to disenroll.[3] Examples of restrictions that could result in favorable selection include preexisting-condition exclusions, higher rates of cost sharing for out-of-plan referrals, restrictions on the use of specialists or choice of hospitals, and narrow interpretations of what is medically necessary.[1,4,5]

In addition to strategies to achieve biased selection that are initiated by health plans, patients themselves can cause bias in enrollment patterns. For example, children with chronic conditions are more likely to have established relationships with providers than children without chronic conditions, and they are more likely to join managed care plans that give them access to those providers. Because children with special health care needs are, on average, more expensive to treat on an annual basis than children without such needs, unless there is an adjustment in the capitation rate for the higher expected cost of caring for these children, health plans that enroll children with special needs will experience what is referred to as adverse selection. Importantly, providers that care for children with chronic conditions, in particular, pediatric subspecialists, are more likely to be financially disadvantaged by an inadequate capitation rate-setting formula than providers whose patient populations are average with regard to health expenditures and health status.

Capitation adjustment methods represent one approach to mitigating the effects of selection bias. These methods can be used to adjust premiums or provider capitation payments to reflect the expected cost of caring for a specific patient population more accurately. Indeed, the Committee on Child Health Financing of the American Academy of Pediatrics has recommended that capitation rates take into account factors such as chronicity and severity of underlying health problems.[6] Several adjustment methods have been identified to accomplish the goal of incorporating a measure of patient health status into the payment system.[7-9] Currently, the options that have been researched can be classified into five generic categories: sociodemographic characteristics, functional health status, clinical indicators, self-reported health status, and prior use.

Basic demographic factors, such as age and gender, are currently used by many Medicaid programs to set payment rates. The major drawback of these and other demographic factors is poor predictive accuracy, because these factors cannot differentiate chronically ill individuals from generally healthy individuals. Of the alternative adjustment methods, most policy and academic interest has focused on prior use of health services as a proxy measure for health status. As an indirect measure of health status, prior use may represent the best predictor of future health costs and use.[8-10] Another important advantage is that most of the data necessary to implement such a system are more readily available than the data needed for survey-based measures.[11] Empirical evidence from published studies confirms the hypothesis that health care use in a previous year, whether measured in terms of prior costs or intensity of prior use, is correlated with subsequent use.[12-14]

Two risk adjustment models based on prior use of hospital services have been developed. The diagnostic cost groups (DCGs) and payment amounts for capitated systems (PACS) both use administrative claims data from inpatient use as a proxy for health status to adjust capitation rates.[15,16] Developed as an alternative to the current rate-setting method for Medicare risk-contracting health maintenance organizations, these methods use an individual's pattern of health care use to predict future expenditures. The predicted expenditures are then used to set capitation payment rates. A third model, the ambulatory care groups (ACGs) case mix system, is based on diagnoses associated with outpatient services.[17] This system seeks to assess a population's "illness burden" to explain variations in the consumption of medical care services, and in contrast to the DCGs and PACS models, ACGs are based on diagnoses associated with ambulatory care services rather than inpatient services.[17,18]

From a pediatric standpoint, a major limitation of the previous research conducted on capitation adjustment, or risk adjustment, is that it has focused primarily on elderly and adult populations.[2,19,20] In fact, most of the research on risk adjustment to date has centered on ways to improve the payment system used by Medicare to reimburse managed care plans serving the elderly.[21,22]

As the number of children enrolled in managed care plans continues to grow, however, the need to develop and test risk adjustment methods on a wider spectrum of age groups becomes more critical. Currently, 44 states and the District of Columbia enroll

Medicaid beneficiaries in managed care plans, with mothers and children comprising most of that enrollment.[23] More than 23% of all Medicaid beneficiaries are enrolled in managed care, and this proportion is expected to increase, as states seek to find innovative approaches to improve access and reduce costs.[24]

Research in the area of pediatric capitation adjustment is especially relevant for children with special health care needs and the providers who care for these children. Without a method for adjusting payment rates to reflect the expected cost of caring for a specific patient population more accurately, health plans can potentially compete on their ability to segment risk rather than on the basis of quality and efficiency.[25] In short, health plans will have a financial incentive to discriminate against children at high risk for greater health expenditures. Providers that attract chronically ill children, such as children's hospitals, also may be disadvantaged, because the patient population that they serve represents children with higher than average health costs. For this reason, health plans may be more reluctant to include them in their provider networks.

The purpose of this study was to take a step toward filling the research gap by testing the predictive performance of current risk adjustment methods on two pediatric populations. A demographic model, an ACG and ambulatory diagnostic group (ADG) model, and an approximation of the DCG and PACS models were tested by using statistical methods similar to those used to develop and test these models. The findings suggest areas in which future development is necessary.

## METHODS

Two data sets were selected for this study, one of which was obtained from the Maryland Medicaid program and the other from the MedCenters Health Plan, a private, nonprofit group model health maintenance organization in Minneapolis, MN, that is now part of the HealthPartners network. Two years (1990 and 1991) of administrative claims data were available from both data sources, and the sample frame for this analysis was limited to children who were continuously enrolled for the entire 2-year study period.

### Dependent Variables

The dependent variable was defined as total health care expenditures in 1991. In the Medicaid population, total expenditures is defined as payments made for all reimbursable services delivered during the year. In the MedCenters population, total health expenditures is defined as gross eligible charges for all covered services. The gross eligible charge field included deductible and copayment amounts. Although paid claims would have been preferable to use than charges, because MedCenters is a managed care plan, this particular field was not available.

Note that these dollar amounts are not equivalent to the actual cost of providing care, nor are they comparable across study populations. Because data from the two populations were not combined, and because the pricing and payment methods for both data sources are consistent from one year to the next, the results should still be meaningful for most audiences.

### Independent Variables

To the greatest extent possible, the independent variables used in this study reflect those used to construct current risk adjustment systems. However, because two of the models, the DCGs and PACS, were developed for use in the Medicare program, not all of the variables are available for a pediatric population. When necessary, proxy variables were assigned or created to serve as appropriate substitutes. Variables used to construct each of the models are described below.

### Demographic Model

The variables used for the demographic model included age and gender. The purpose of constructing a model based on demographic factors was to replicate the current method that is typically used by most Medicaid programs to set payment rates. As a standard, the demographic model offers a useful comparison against which the other, more complex models can be assessed.

### DCG Model

The variables that make up the DCG model include age, gender, welfare status, and DCG category.[21] A patient's DCG category is based on the primary diagnosis associated with hospitalizations lasting 3 days or longer occurring during a base period. The diagnostic information is used to categorize patients into one of nine DCGs, which were developed by using diagnosis and cost data from the Medicare population. A base period of 12 months is generally needed to assign DCGs, and patients with more than one hospitalization in that period are grouped into the highest DCG category.[16]

Because of data constraints and programmatic differences, we could not replicate DCGs completely. Welfare status was not included as a variable for this study, because one study population, Maryland Medicaid, is composed primarily of children who qualify for welfare, whereas the other population, the MedCenters health plan, did not enroll Medicaid beneficiaries at the time the data were collected. In addition, although age was included as a categorical variable in the original DCG model, here it is included as a continuous variable, primarily for comparability purposes with the other risk adjustment models and also because the age categories specified for DCGs are for an elderly population.

### PACS Model

Like the DCGs, the PACS model was intended to serve as an alternative to the current Medicare payment method.[15] The health status factors included in the PACS model are: age, gender, prior disability entitlement, number of admissions in each major diagnostic category (MDC), number of discharges by level of chronicity (chronic, acute, or acute with sequelae), whether a patient had zero, one, or more than one hospitalization in the base period, and whether the Medicare part B deductible was met.[22]

Because the Medicaid program does not charge an out-of-pocket deductible for outpatient services, and the expenditure variable in the MedCenters data includes copayments and deductibles, a proxy variable was established for the variable indicating whether the Medicare ambulatory deductible was met. The proxy is a dummy variable indicating whether total ambulatory costs for a child exceeded $75 in 1990, which is the equivalent of the Medicare deductible in 1984 when the PACS model was developed.

In the case of MDCs, we found that for several categories the numbers of cases were not adequate enough for meaningful analysis. To address this problem, 11 MDC categories were combined on the basis of clinical comparability to create 5 new modified categories. These include: MDC3_4, MDC3 (ear, nose, mouth, and throat) and MDC4 (respiratory system); MDC13_15, MDC13 (female reproductive system), MDC14 (pregnancy, childbirth, and puerperium), and MDC15 (newborns and other neonates); MDC16_17, MDC16 (blood and blood-forming organs and immunologic disorders) and MDC17 (myeloproliferative diseases and poorly differentiated neoplasms); MDC19_20, MDC19 (mental disease and disorders) and MDC20 (alcohol and drug use and alcohol- and drug-induced organic mental disorders); and MDC21_22, MDC21 (poisonings and toxic effects of drugs) and MDC22 (burns).

### ACG Model

The ACG case mix system is different from the risk adjustment models described above because it is based on diagnoses associated with ambulatory care services rather than inpatient services.[17] Patients are categorized into 1 of 51 ACGs based on their age, gender, and diagnosis codes of the International Classification of Diseases, ninth revision (ICD-9), clinical modification, incurred during a defined period of time in an ambulatory setting. To assign a patient to a specific ACG category, all diagnosis codes are grouped into 1 of 34 clinically similar ADGs. Although the ACGs are mutually exclusive categories, patients can have an unlimited number of combinations of ADGs, because individuals with more than one diagnosis during the given time period will probably fall into more than one ADG.

Because of the analytical difference between the ACGs and the ADGs, it is possible to construct two separate models. Thus, the independent variables in the first model are age, gender, and the 34 ADG categories, and the second model includes each of the 51 ACG cells. Because age and gender already are incorporated into the ACGs, they are not included as independent variables in the model.

### Individual Level Analysis

Multiple linear regression, or ordinary least squares, was used to test the predictive performance of each risk adjustment model at the individual level on a prospective basis. The dependent variable was total expenditures in 1991, and the independent variables were calculated by using 1990 data. Like many of the previous studies on risk adjustment, predictive performance was measured by the adjusted $R^2$ statistic.[9,11,21,26] The adjusted $R^2$ is one measure of goodness of fit and can be interpreted as the percentage of variability in the dependent variable that is explained by the set of independent variables in the model.

When expressed as a percentage, the $R^2$ value can range from 0% to 100%. However, in actuality no model could possibly predict 100% of the health expenditures in a population. The maximum explainable variance is affected by the proportion of health expenditures that results from random illnesses, injuries, and health events that cannot be predicted.[2] Indeed, the goal is to be able to explain only enough variance so that risk selection will not occur.

### Split-half Validation Using Randomly Selected Groups

Cross-validation of the selected risk adjustment models was performed by using a split-half method.[27,28] The split-half method applied in this study involved the random partitioning of the data into two halves. The first half of the data was used to develop the model and to determine coefficient weights. Like the analysis conducted at the individual level, the models were developed by using total expenditures in 1991 as the dependent variable and the alternative risk adjustment factors as independent variables.

Predictive performance for the split-half analysis is determined by using a predictive ratio, which is equal to the average predicted expenditures divided by the average actual expenditures. The closer this value comes to 1.0, the better the performance of the model for that population. An example of how predicted values were calculated can be found in "Appendix."

### Split-half Validation Using Nonrandom Groups

In addition to randomly selected groups, the models also were tested by using two groups that were intentionally selected to represent children at higher or lower than average risk for greater future resource use, or nonrandom. For this analysis, predictor weights were derived from the estimation half and applied to selected subsamples from the validation half.

The first nonrandom group was composed of children with one or more chronic conditions and was intended to represent children at higher than average risk for greater expenditures. These children were identified by using version 3.0 of the Classification of Congenital and Chronic Child Health Conditions that was developed by the National Association of Children's Hospitals and Related Institutions.

This list of conditions, which contains approximately 2500 ICD-9 codes at the five-digit level, accounts for an appreciable proportion of the patient population in children's hospitals. The diagnosis codes in both data sets were cross-matched against the ICD-9 codes occurring on the list. For the split-half analysis that was conducted by using this particular selection method, only children whose diagnosis codes matched with the National Association of Children's Hospitals and Related Institutions list were selected for the validation half of the data.

The second nonrandom group was based on children who were identified as nonusers of health care services in the first year. These children had no health expenditures in 1990. Like the analysis based on children with chronic conditions for the split-half analysis that was conducted with this particular method, only children who did not incur any health expenditures in the first year were selected from the validation half.

## RESULTS

### Individual Level Results

Table 1 displays the adjusted $R^2$ results for the demographic model and the four basic risk adjustment methods. These results clearly suggest that any of the alternative capitation adjustment methods perform better than a demographic model that includes only age and gender. These demographic factors were able to explain less than 0.1% of the variance in expenditures in either study population. The PACS model performed better than all other models in both populations, with adjusted $R^2$s of 10.67% and 7.22% in the Medicaid and MedCenters populations, respectively.

### Group Level Regression Results

For the split-half validation in which the validation data set comprised randomly selected children, all models performed comparably well (Table 2). The results show that a demographic model would overpay managed care plans by 2% in the Medicaid population and would underpay plans by 1% in the MedCenters population, relative to the amount currently paid. The predictive ratios for all five models are close to 1.0, although the Medicaid results seem to be greater than 1.0, and the MedCenters results tend to be slightly less.

### Group Level Results Based on Nonrandom Groups

Because an enrolled population rarely reflects a random sample from a given risk pool, findings from the split-half validation using nonrandomly selected groups are particularly important. Table 3 displays results for the split-half analysis in which the validation data set was limited to children with one or more chronic conditions.

Although any of the other four models offer an improvement over the demographic model, significant underpayment would still result for high-risk patients. The demographic model would pay a managed care plan, on average, only 24% of the actual cost of enrolling a child with a chronic illness in the

**TABLE 1.** Adjusted $R^2$ for Prospective Models

| Risk Adjustment Model | Adjusted $R^2$, %* | |
|---|---|---|
| | Maryland Medicaid (n = 87 793) | MedCenters (n = 45 765) |
| Demographics | 0.07 | 0.00 |
| Diagnostic cost groups | 5.32 | 6.06 |
| Ambulatory diagnosis groups | 7.30 | 4.14 |
| Ambulatory care groups | 5.28 | 2.52 |
| Payment amounts for capitated systems | 10.67 | 7.22 |

* The adjusted $R^2$ is the proportion of variance in total expenditures that is explained by the set of independent variables, in this case the variables in each of the risk adjustment models. The $R^2$ values displayed here are expressed in percentages, and as such, the maximum value that could be obtained is 100%.

**TABLE 2.** Predictive Performance Measures for Split-half Validation

| Risk Adjustment Model | Predictive Ratio* | |
|---|---|---|
| | Maryland Medicaid (n = 43 897) | MedCenters (n = 22 888) |
| Demographics | 1.02 | 0.99 |
| Diagnostic cost groups | 1.04 | 0.98 |
| Ambulatory diagnosis groups | 1.02 | 1.01 |
| Ambulatory care groups | 1.03 | 1.00 |
| Payment amounts for capitated systems | 1.03 | 0.99 |

* The predictive ratio is equal to the average predicted expenditures divided by the average actual expenditures. The closer this value comes to 1.0, the better the performance of the model for that population. Values less than 1.0 indicate underprediction or underpayment, and values greater than 1.0 indicate overprediction or overpayment.

**TABLE 3.** Predictive Performance Measures for Split-half Validation: Where Validation Data Set Includes Only Children With Chronic Conditions

| Risk Adjustment Model | Predictive Ratio* | |
|---|---|---|
| | Maryland Medicaid (n = 5 684) | MedCenters (n = 119) |
| Demographics | 0.24 | 0.06 |
| Diagnostic cost groups | 0.44 | 0.41 |
| Ambulatory diagnosis groups | 0.82 | 0.25 |
| Ambulatory care groups | 0.69 | 0.17 |
| Payment amounts for capitated systems | 0.62 | 0.44 |

* The predictive ratio is equal to the average predicted expenditures divided by the average actual expenditures. The closer this value comes to 1.0, the better the performance of the model for that population. Values less than 1.0 indicate underprediction or underpayment, and values greater than 1.0 indicate overprediction or overpayment.

Medicaid program and only 6% in the MedCenters program. For the ADG model, which performed better than the other models in the Medicaid data, the difference between predicted and actual resource use for chronically ill children enrolled in a Medicaid managed care program would be 18%. The PACS model, which performed best in the MedCenters population, would pay only 44% of the actual cost. This amount indicates how much participating plans could lose, on average, when they enroll a child with a chronic health condition. Consequently, implementation of any of these methods would not necessarily eliminate the incentive for selection bias.

Just as a health plan could lose money by enrolling high-risk children, they could also gain by enrolling children representing lower-than-average risk. A demographic model would pay 418% more than the actual cost of enrolling a child in the Medicaid program who did not use any medical services in the previous year (Table 4). Thus, although the risk adjustment models are more likely to underpredict expenditures for high-risk children, they are more likely to overpredict for low-risk children. The exception to this trend was the ADG model in the MedCenters population.

**TABLE 4.** Predictive Performance Measures for Split-half Validation: Where Validation Data Set Includes Only Children Who Were Nonusers in 1990

| Risk Adjustment Model | Predictive Ratio* | |
| --- | --- | --- |
| | Maryland Medicaid (n = 11 423) | MedCenters (n = 2 386) |
| Demographics | 5.18 | 2.83 |
| Diagnostic cost groups | 4.25 | 2.62 |
| Ambulatory diagnosis groups | 1.53 | 0.53 |
| Ambulatory care groups | 1.35 | 1.40 |
| Payment amounts for capitated systems | 1.60 | 1.32 |

* The predictive ratio is equal to the average predicted expenditures divided by the average actual expenditures. The closer this value comes to 1.0, the better the performance of the model for that population. Values less than 1.0 indicate underprediction or underpayment, and values greater than 1.0 indicate overprediction or overpayment.

## DISCUSSION

Proposed methods to address the problem of risk selection include regulation, reinsurance, and risk adjustment. Each of these approaches addresses a different aspect of risk segmentation, and each has inherent advantages and limitations. Importantly, these methods are not necessarily mutually exclusive and can be used together in a combined approach.

A number of procompetitive regulatory measures aimed at reducing selection bias on the part of health plans have been proposed.[29-31] Guaranteed issue and renewal of health insurance, prohibiting preexisting condition exclusions and waiting periods, and establishing a monitoring mechanism for those who disenroll or switch health plans are examples of such legislation. Alone, however, these measures are not likely to eliminate selection bias, primarily because this type of regulation addresses explicit practices rather than more subtle ones, such as limiting access to specialty referrals.[32,33] Moreover, state regulations do not apply to the ever-expanding self-insured population that is covered by the federal Employee Retirement Income Security Act (ERISA) of 1974.[34]

Retrospective reinsurance, a second method that has been identified to limit the effects of selection bias, would require health plans in a given market to pay into a risk pool. For large claims greater than a set dollar amount or outlier threshold, plans would be reimbursed out of the pool for a proportion of these high-cost claims.[35] New York State has established an alternative to this approach based on specific diagnoses rather than claims exceeding a certain dollar threshold. Under this arrangement, a pool for organ transplants, low birth weight infants, patients with acquired immunodeficiency syndrome, and ventilator-dependent patients has been established.[36] The disadvantage of a reinsurance approach is that health plans lose the difference between the actual payment and the threshold amount for every child above the threshold. This creates a financial incentive not to enroll these patients. Furthermore, the disease-specific approach does not protect children who have conditions other than those that are explicitly covered.

Risk adjustment, or capitation adjustment, represents a third approach to addressing the issue of selection bias. The fundamental principle behind capitation adjustment is the inclusion of health-related characteristics of enrolled populations into the payment system to achieve fair and adequate rates.[7,8] Without adjusting rates to reflect the expected cost of caring for a specific patient population more accurately, health plans will compete on their ability to segment risk rather than on the basis of quality and efficiency.[25] And ultimately, biased selection based on the nonrandom assignment of health risks can undermine a health care reform model that relies on competition to control costs. To ensure efficiency and maintain access to care for patients representing higher risk, rates should be set so that low-risk plans or providers are not overpaid and high-risk plans or providers are not unfairly penalized.[37]

The methods tested in this study are classified as prior use models. In addition to receiving the most policy and academic interest, prior use has also received the most scrutiny. There are valid concerns with all prior use models. Among the criticisms is that prior use measures create a financial incentive to provide services in the current year to raise the capitation rate in the subsequent year.[38] Managed care organizations in particular contend that payment systems based on prior use would penalize plans that have successfully controlled the use rates of their enrollees by paying them a lower capitation amount.[39] Some have argued that prior use models would eventually result in experience-rated capitation rates, which would be the equivalent of a cost-based system with a 1-year lag.[10] In addition, others suggest that data systems vary between indemnity plans and managed care plans, and that this factor could make risk adjustment based on claims data complex and difficult to implement.[19,40] Availability of data would be a problem for new enrollees and other groups lacking prior use data, such as infants.

Despite these concerns, claims-based prior use models are more likely to be adopted than the alternatives. These measures have demonstrated equal or better performance than any of the other measures with respect to predictive accuracy.[9] Furthermore, for plans that currently collect and maintain administrative claims data, these data are more convenient and accessible than survey data. More importantly for pediatric capitation adjustment, survey-based measures, such as functional health status, perceived health status, and clinical descriptors, are not readily available or may be inappropriate for children. They are also expensive to collect and are affected by nonresponse bias.[41]

Results from this study indicate that, at the individual level, each of the risk adjustment models was able to explain a greater proportion of the variance in total health expenditures than a demographic model based on age and gender. The model based on age and gender, which is currently the most common method used to set payment rates by Medicaid and other insurers, was able to explain less than 0.1% of the variance in expenditures for either population. The other models were able to explain between 2.5%

and 10.7% of the variance. The predictive performance of the PACS model was higher than that for the other models in both populations. In the Maryland Medicaid population the ADG model also performed well (adjusted $R^2$ = 7.30%). and in the Med-Centers population the DCG model performed well (adjusted $R^2$ = 6.06%).

To some readers the amount of variance explained by these models may seem relatively small. However, only a limited proportion of total variance is actually predictable. A substantial proportion of health care expenditures results from random illnesses, injuries, and health events that cannot be predicted.[42] For example, one study determined that the maximum explainable variance in total ambulatory expenditures for children is only 37%.[2] Indeed, it is the risk and uncertainty associated with random health events that compels us to purchase insurance.[43] Unlike chronic illnesses, random events will not necessarily lead to risk selection or access problems if health plans or providers are paid an average amount of these expenditures. The objective of capitation adjustment is to be able to explore the predictable amount. The fact that only a proportion of the variance in expenditures is actually explainable suggests that additional work is necessary.

In addition to the individual level analysis, we report here on the results from a split-half validation to assess the performance of the models at a group level. For the randomly selected group, the demographic model performed as well as any of the other more sophisticated risk adjustment measures. The predictive ratios were comparable for all models and across both data sets.

A reasonable conclusion to make, based on these findings, is that if the distribution of health risks across plans or provider groups were truly random, risk adjustment methods might not be necessary. However, health risk is seldom distributed uniformly across enrolled populations, with some plans and providers having favorable selection and others having adverse selection. For this reason, the split-half validation performed on randomly selected data is not likely to reflect actual enrollment patterns in situations in which individuals can select from among competing health plans and may overestimate the performance of the models in a real-world setting.

Because the purpose of developing and implementing capitation adjustment methods is to protect patients and providers from the effects of biased selection, it was crucial that each of the adjustment methods be tested on nonrandom groups. The split-half validation using nonrandom groups accomplished this goal. Findings from the group comprising children with one or more chronic conditions indicate that all of the models were able to predict expenditures better than the demographic model, although substantial underprediction remained. Conversely, for the low-risk group, represented by children who did not incur any health care expenses in the first year, nearly all of the models overpredicted future expenditures.

Several limitations of this study should be noted.

First, the use of paid claims in the Medicaid population and gross eligible charges in the MedCenters population are not necessarily accurate measures of the true costs associated with providing health care services.[44,45] For example, evidence suggests that Medicaid reimbursement to physicians for pediatric care under Medicaid is inadequate.[46] Consequently, the component of total expenditures represented by physician services may underestimate the actual cost of providing care. With regard to the MedCenters health plan, as is the case with many arrangements between private health plans and provider networks, payment rates and discounts are negotiated with provider groups and hospitals, meaning that gross eligible charges also may not be indicative of true costs.[44,45] Furthermore, charges for private insurers in general may be greater than actual costs because of cost shifting by providers.[45]

Despite these caveats, paid claims and charges are used as estimates of resource use in this study. Because data from the two populations were not combined, and the pricing and payment methods for both data sources are consistent from one year to the next, the results should still be meaningful for most audiences. Thus, although the dollar amounts reported here are not necessarily equivalent to the actual cost of providing care, they reflect actual amounts paid by the Maryland Medicaid program and the MedCenters health plan.

Children who were not continuously enrolled for the entire study period were excluded from this analysis. Partial-year enrollment can occur when enrollees join or disenroll from the plan and also because of births and deaths. In the Medicaid program, partial-year enrollment also can result from changes in eligibility that occur throughout the year. For example, children can gain, lose, and regain eligibility during the course of a year. Moreover, limiting the sample frame to children who were continuously enrolled means that infants and neonates were not included in the analysis. Infants with severe birth defects and infants who were born prematurely can be substantially more expensive to care for than infants without such problems.

The practical issues that partial-year enrollees represent are complex and were beyond the scope of this study. However, excluding partial-year enrollees from the sample frame represents an important limitation of this study, because a fair and equitable rate-setting method must adjust for these children. On the other hand, children who were not enrolled for an entire year are likely to be different from those who were, and including them in the denominator could potentially have affected results of the study.

Another important qualification to note is that the DCG model, more than the other models, suffered from the effects of testing a system that was designed for an entirely different population. The diagnosis and cost information used to create the DCG categories was based exclusively on Medicare data and was not intended for use in other populations. This fact makes testing the model with a pediatric population susceptible to a host of conceptual and technical problems.

In conclusion, rate setting based on demographic

factors is inadequate in predicting future resource use for children. Limitations associated with current alternatives, however, suggest the need for further research to develop and test pediatric risk adjusters. Results from this study indicate that the findings are inconsistent; some models perform better than others under certain circumstances, whereas other models perform better under other circumstances. No single method emerged as a clear choice. One approach might be to construct a combined model that incorporates the strongest predictor variables from each of the methods. However, further research is needed to confirm the appropriateness of this method and to identify which variables demonstrate consistency across various populations.

Without risk adjustment, health plans could potentially compete on their ability to segment risk rather than on the basis of quality and efficiency. And without a capitation adjustment system that can be applied to pediatric populations, health plans will have a financial incentive to discriminate against children at high risk for greater health expenditures. For children with chronic conditions, findings at both the individual and group levels suggest that any of the current risk adjustment methods would still leave chronically ill children at risk of discrimination in a competitive health care market. In other words, the disincentive to enroll children with costly conditions and special health care needs would not be eliminated by any of the capitation adjustment methods tested in this study.

Moreover, without adequate capitation adjustment methods, providers that care for chronically ill children, such as pediatric subspecialists and children's hospitals, may be financially disadvantaged because their patient populations represent children with higher-than-average health costs. For these providers the bottom line is that one size does not fit all with regard to capitation adjustment methods.

## ACKNOWLEDGMENTS

This project was supported by grant R03 HS08441 from the Agency for Health Care Policy and Research as part of its dissertation grant program.

We gratefully acknowledge the assistance of Jonathan Weiner, Neil Powe, and Bernard Guyer, all of whom provided helpful insight into this study. In addition, we are grateful to the National Association of Children's Hospitals and Related Institutions for permission to use an earlier version of their classification of childhood health conditions.

## APPENDIX

Predicted total expenditures (TOTEXP) were calculated as follows, using the demographic model as an example. A multiple linear regression model was constructed, which can be written as:

$$TOTEXP = \alpha + \beta_{age}(AGE) + \beta_{sex}(SEX) + e$$

The $\beta$ coefficients $\beta_{age}$ and $\beta_{sex}$ were then applied to the second half of the data set to determine expected values. Specifically, the expected values, or predicted costs (PRED), were calculated for each child, $i$, by multiplying the child's age by $\beta_{age}$, multiplying gen-

der by $\beta_{sex}$, and summing the amounts together with the intercept:

$$PRED_i = \alpha + \beta_{age}(AGE_i) + \beta_{sex}(SEX_i)$$

Predicted costs for the sample were obtained by aggregating the predicted amount for each child in the sample, and this process was repeated for both data sets. Model performance was evaluated by comparing predicted expenditures with actual expenditures divided by the average of the actual expenditures. The closer the predictive ratio comes to 1.0, the better the performance of the model for that population.

## REFERENCES

1. Schlesinger M, Mechanic D. Challenges for managed competition from chronic illness. *Health Aff (Millwood).* 1993;12:123–137
2. Newhouse JP, Sloss EM, Manning WG, Keeler EB. Risk adjustment for a children's capitation rate. *Health Care Finance Rev.* 1993;15:39–54
3. Wrightson CW. *HMO Rate Setting Financial Strategy.* Ann Arbor, MI: Health Administration Press Perspective; 1990
4. Lichtenstein R, Thomas JW, Watkins B, et al. HMO marketing and selection bias: are TEFRA HMOs skimming? *Med Care.* 1992;30:329–346
5. Fox HB, Wicks LB, Newacheck PW. Health maintenance organizations and children with special health care needs. *Am J Dis Child.* 1993;147: 546–552
6. Committee on Child Health Financing. Guiding principles for managed care arrangements for the health care of infants, children, adolescents, and young adults. *Pediatrics.* 1995;95:613–615
7. Thomas JW, Lichtenstein R, Wyszewianski L, Berki SE. Increasing Medicare enrollment in HMOs: the need for capitation rates adjusted for health status. *Inquiry.* 1983;20:227–239
8. Lubitz J. Health status adjustments for Medicare capitation. *Inquiry.* 1987;24:362–375
9. Epstein AM, Cumella EJ. Capitation payment: using predictors of medical utilization to adjust rates. *Health Care Finance Rev.* 1988;10:51–69
10. Thomas JW, Lichtenstein R. Including health status in Medicare's adjusted average per capita cost capitation formula. *Med Care.* 1986;24: 259–275
11. Beebe J, Lubitz J, Eggers P. Using prior utilization to determine payments for Medicare enrollees in health maintenance organizations. *Health Care Finance Rev.* 1985;6:27–38
12. McCall N, Wai HS. An analysis of the use of Medicare services by the continuously enrolled aged. *Med Care.* 1983;21:567–585
13. Lubitz J, Beebe J, Riley G. Improving the Medicare HMO payment formula to deal with biased selection. *Adv Health Econ Health Serv Res.* 1985;6:101–122
14. Eggers P, Prihoda R. Preenrollment reimbursement patterns of Medicare beneficiaries enrolled in "at risk" HMOs. *Health Care Finance Rev.* 1982;4:55–73
15. Anderson GF, Lupu D, Powe N, et al. *Payment Amounts for Capitated Systems.* Baltimore, MD: The Johns Hopkins University; 1989. Health Care Financing Administration report 17-C-98990/3
16. Ellis RP, Ash A. *Refining the Diagnostic Cost Group Model: A Proposed Modification to the AAPCC for HMO Reimbursement.* Boston, MA: Boston University; 1988. Health Care Financing Administration report 18-C-98526/1-03
17. Weiner JP, Starfield BH, Steinwachs DM, et al. Development and application of a population-oriented measure of ambulatory care case mix. *Med Care.* 1991;29:452–472
18. Starfield B, Weiner J, Mumford L, et al. Ambulatory care groups: a categorization of diagnoses for research and management. *Health Serv Res.* 1991;26:53–74
19. Hornbrook MC, Goodman MJ, Bennett MD, Greenlick MR. Assessing health plan case mix in employed populations: self-reported health status models. *Adv Health Econ Health Serv Res.* 1991;12:233–272
20. Robinson JC, Luft HS, Gardner LB, Morrison EM. A method of risk-adjusting employer contributions to competing health insurance plans. *Inquiry.* 1991;28:107–116
21. Ash A, Porell F, Gruenberg L, et al. Adjusting Medicare capitation payments using prior hospitalization data. *Health Care Finance Rev.* 1989;10:17–29
22. Anderson GF, Steinberg EP, Powe NR, et al. Setting payment rates for capitated systems: a comparison of various alternatives. *Inquiry.* 1990; 27:225–233

23. Riley T. Medicaid: the role of the states. *JAMA*. 1995;274:267–270
24. Rowland D. Medicaid at 30: new challenges for the nation's health safety net. *JAMA*. 1995;274:271–273
25. Luft HS, Miller RH. Patient selection in a competitive health care system. *Health Aff (Millwood)*. 1988;7:97–119
26. van Vliet RC, van De Ven WP. Capitation payments based on prior hospitalizations. *Health Econ*. 1993;2:177–188
27. Picard RR, Cook D. Cross-validation of regression models. *J Am Stat Assoc*. 1984;79:575–583
28. Snee RD. Validation of regression models: methods and examples. *Technometrics*. 1977;19:415–428
29. Moore M. *Risk Adjustment Under Managed Competition*. Jackson Hole, WY: Jackson Hole Group; 1993
30. Congressional Budget Office. *Managed Competition and Its Potential to Reduce Health Spending*. Washington, DC: US Government Printing Office; 1993
31. Health Policy Alternatives, Inc. *Managed Competition and Other Health Reform Proposals*. Washington, DC: Health Policy Alternatives, Inc; 1993. Report prepared for the Health Care Technology Institute
32. Newhouse JP. Patients at risk: health reform and risk adjustment. *Health Aff (Millwood)*. 1994;13:132–146
33. Steinmetz G. Clinton health plan skirts issue of bias by insurers against riskier customers. *The Wall Street Journal*. September 14, 1993:B8
34. Wehr E, Jameson EJ. Beyond benefits: the importance of a pediatric standard in private insurance contracts to ensuring health care access for children. *Future of Children*. 1994;4:115–133
35. White House Task Force on Health Risk Pooling. *Health Risk Pooling for Small-Group Health Insurance*. Washington, DC: White House Task Force on Health Risk Pooling; 1993
36. New York Department of Insurance. *Establishment and Operation of Market Stabilization Mechanisms for Individual and Small Group Health Insurance and Medicare Supplement Insurance*. New York, NY: New York Department of Insurance; 1992. Regulation 146
37. Hornbrook MC, Bennett MD, Greenlick MR. Adjusting the AAPCC for selectivity and selection bias under Medicare risk contracts. *Adv Health Econ Health Serv Res*. 1989;10:111–149
38. McClure W. On the research status of risk-adjusted capitation rates. *Inquiry*. 1984;21:205–213
39. Hornbrook MC, Goodman MJ. Health plan case mix: definition, measurement, and use. *Adv Health Econ Health Serv Res*. 1991;12:111–148
40. Hornbrook MC, Greenlick MR, Bennett MD, Goodman MJ. *Self-Reported Health Status Risk Adjusters for the Medicare AAPCC Based on an HMO's Experience*. Portland, OR: Kaiser Permanente Center for Health Research; 1991. Health Care Financing Administration report 18-C-98804-1/04
41. Park Nicollet Medical Foundation. *A Comparison of Alternative Approaches to Risk Measurement*. Minneapolis, MN: Health Research Center; 1994. Physician Payment Review Commission report 93-G07
42. Newhouse JP, Manning WG, Keeler EB, Sloss EM. Adjusting capitation rates using objective health measures and prior utilization. *Health Care Finance Rev*. 1989;10:41–54
43. Jacobs P. *The Economics of Health and Medical Care*. Gaithersburg, MD: Aspen Publishers, Inc; 1991
44. Lave JR, Pashos CL, Anderson GF, et al. Costing medical care: using Medicare administrative data. *Med Care*. 1994;32:JS77-JS89
45. Finkler SA. The distinction between cost and charges. *Ann Intern Med*. 1982;96:102–109
46. McManus M, Flint S, Kelly R. The adequacy of physician reimbursement for pediatric care under Medicaid. *Pediatrics*. 1991;87:909–920

# OTHER AAP
# RESOURCES

# Physicians: What Parents Want You to Know About Their Child With Special Needs

## THE PARENT'S POINT OF VIEW

### I Like You When You:

- Recognize my denial, anger, and healthy and natural response to grief.
- Accept that my child's health care needs are only a part of my family's priorities and that some-times my family's needs and concerns may take precedence.
- Value that I'm the expert on my child.
- Acknowledge that I am a compe-tent partner in health care.

### What I Need From You:

- Help me find the information I need to understand my child's condition. My child's condition is not temporary. I'll be learning about it for a lifetime.
- Do not withhold or omit any information concerning the severity or extent of my child's condition. Also, do not hesitate to use medical terms when necessary.
- Help me to understand the range of possibilities. Tell me the worst and best possible prognosis.
- Acknowledge my sense of urgency by responding quickly to requests for medical information, referrals, etc, so that appropriate services can begin or continue.
- Remind me of my child's strengths from time to time.

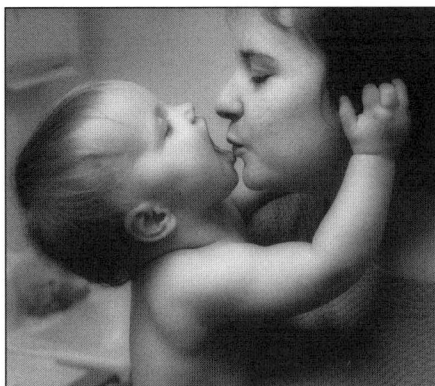

- Collaborate with other pro-fessionals providing care for my child.

If it sometimes seems I expect you to be my social worker, psychiatrist, and omnipotent seer of the future... well I do!

### P.S. Thanks for being my competent partner in health care!

The American Academy of Pediatrics (AAP) believes that all infants, children, adolescents, and young adults should have access to a "medical home" that provides comprehensive, coordinated, and family-centered health care.

This goal presents unique challenges for pediatricians offering primary health care to children with special needs within this changing health delivery system. To meet those challenges, the Medical Home Program for Children With Special

Needs identifies and promotes model strategies, training, and technical assistance. By supporting physicians, and other health care professionals, the Medical Home Program for Children With Special Needs seeks to provide better health care for all children.

For more information on how the Medical Home Program for Children With Special Needs can be a resource for you, or if you would like to be added to the mailing list, contact Liz Osterhus, AAP Department of Community Pediatrics, 800/433-9016, ext 7621.

*Parent-professional collaboration is an essential component in the provision of medical homes for children with special needs. This document was brought to you by the American Academy of Pediatrics, Medical Home Program for Children With Special Needs with funding provided by the federal Maternal and Child Health Bureau.*

*This document is a reprint from materials provided by the Hawaii Medical Associa-tion's former Medical Home Project.*

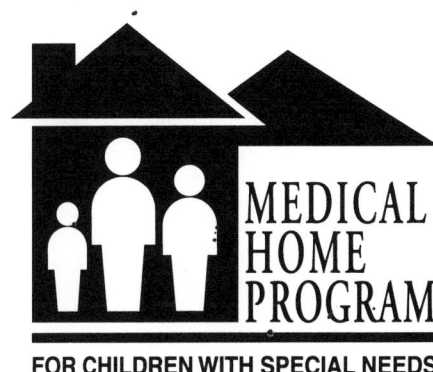

**MEDICAL HOME PROGRAM**

**FOR CHILDREN WITH SPECIAL NEEDS**

# SPECIAL RESOURCES FOR SPECIAL CHILDREN

## The Medical Home and Early Intervention: Linking Services for Children With Special Needs

Special needs call for specialized education, not only for patients and their families but also for the professionals who support them. This 16-page handbook serves as a unique resource for child advocates to promote a continuum of care for young children with special health care needs. The text focuses on two major components of the continuum of care:

- The provision of community-based health services through the concept of the medical home

- The role of the Early Intervention Program for Infants and Toddlers With Disabilities in providing the statewide system for early intervention services

A joint effort of the AAP Medical Home Program for Children With Special Health Care Needs and the federal Maternal and Child Health Bureau, *The Medical Home and Early Intervention* is useful for anyone involved in early intervention services for young children with special needs (birth through age 3 years).

For more information on obtaining this handbook, call the AAP Department of Publications at 800/433-9016.

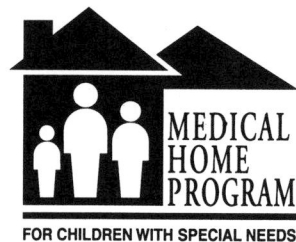

MEDICAL HOME PROGRAM
FOR CHILDREN WITH SPECIAL NEEDS

# ADDITIONAL MANAGED CARE MATERIALS

Healthcare is changing with amazing speed. While you are keeping up with breakthroughs in technology and treatment, don't neglect managed care and its implications for your practice. We can help you meet the challenge.

*A Pediatrician's Guide to Managed Care,* a resource from the American Academy of Pediatrics, features practical information that explains how to maximize strategies and minimize risk in the new healthcare environment.

After defining managed care and discussing it from a public and private perspective, this resource guide concentrates on the details. When you finish reading, you'll understand:

- Current models, including HMOs, PPOs, POS, and integrated delivery systems
- Assessing capitation rates and understanding carve-outs and exclusions
- Managed care organization assessment
- Negotiating managed care contracts
- Legal and antitrust issues related to negotiation and organizations
- Issues related to selling your practice
- Implications for pediatric specialists, and children with special needs and their parents

To clarify complex issues, *A Pediatrician's Guide to Managed Care* includes a glossary of terms, the AAP Policy Statement on Managed Care and the Antitrust Policy, and CPT and ICD-9-CM codes for pediatric services and, to get hands-on practice, you will also find a practice and contract checklist.

*How to Use Your Managed Care Plan Effectively: Questions and Answers for Families With Children* is a must for families enrolled in managed care plans and pediatricians who want to instruct families. Questions cover such topics as accessing pediatric primary and specialty providers and children's hospitals, understanding authorization for care, linking with other child and family services in the community, cost-sharing requirements, accessing out-of-plan or out-of-area services, and plan exclusions and limitations.

*Purchasing Quality Pediatric Care in Commercial Managed Care Plans* is designed to educate health care purchasers, including corporate benefit officers, health care benefit consultants, and state legislators, on the need to include comprehensive quality pediatric health care services in all managed care plans. This brochure describes unique pediatric features to look for in benefit plans, provider networks, and quality improvement mechanisms.

Look for additional reports on emerging managed care issues published three times a year in *AAP News.* Future issues will concentrate on selling a practice, special needs children and managed care, and the concerns of hospital-based providers with regards to managed care including a discussion of advanced capitation methodologies.

**Managed Care Slide Kit.** The ramifications of managed care are affecting pediatricians in every area. *The best plan for the future is one* *based on knowledge.* Therefore the American Academy of Pediatrics brings you ongoing strategies for managed care. Our latest resource is the Managed Care Slide Kit. Based on the highly successful publication, *A Pediatrician's Guide to Managed Care*, this slide presentation focuses on managed care models, reimbursement options, and negotiating a managed care contract.

The *59 slides and an accompanying script* can be used as:

An **educational tool** to educate health professionals on the changing nature of managed care.

A **speaker's aid** for making presentations at local health coalitions, resident groups, hospital medical staff meetings, or other forums where it is important to get the message out regarding pediatricians and managed care.

For more information on obtaining these Managed Care materials, call the AAP Department of Publications at 800/433-9016.